# Beyond Right and Wrong

Introductory Medical Ethics for Students and Junior
Practitioners

# Introduction

Everyone in the field of medicine faces ethical dilemmas. That is not up for debate. From routine clinical discussions to policy decisions to critical end-of-life choices and beyond, everyone from the doctors and nurses to the technicians and healthcare assistants is faced with ethical dilemmas. Some may think such issues are unimportant and easily resolved from their perspectives or simply beyond their immediate job description. Or perhaps you, the reader, see the complexity of such dilemmas as overwhelming and impossible even to approach. Or perhaps you still think such dilemmas are not your problem and are the purview of senior doctors alone or some dedicated ethics committee. Yet, each person on the medical team has a role to play, and medical ethics does not discriminate between job titles. If you are a health science student, you will face such dilemmas soon, and your voice will matter. If you are already a healthcare team member, the dilemmas are already in front of you, assuming you pay attention.

The last few years have seen a substantial shift in the attitudes of many peoples in societies worldwide. The values and principles guiding professionals, previously taken for granted, are increasingly threatened by social, religious, and political ideologies, which may undermine the quality of care that all in the healthcare field are committed to providing. The field of medical ethics is comparatively young in the context of medical education and medical practice. Furthermore, it is often taught in a manner that, despite teachers' best efforts, fails to convey the importance of the foundational values of the practice of medicine. This may be because of intrinsic biases within the course, institution, or geopolitical context and reliance on 'traditional' models of medical education. Further, ethics is often underemphasized and even entirely untaught in some curricula. It may instead be moral philosophy, legal medicine, theology or deontology, none of which teach you how to think, but instead to outsource dilemmas and debate to seniors, religious figures, academics, and politicians.

In planning the writing of this book, part of the inspiration was to formulate a text which would encourage students and practitioners alike to move beyond the moral confines of yesteryears and provide the tools and foundations to produce the clinical ethics of tomorrow. In moving beyond deontological codes and legal frameworks, we may reach an equivalent of the moral evolution postulated by Nietzsche in his book "Beyond Good and Evil". Nevertheless, it would be beyond arrogant to present this as an equivalent work (or even in the same ballpark). Still, hopefully, it may be a starting point, the first steppingstone of sorts, towards a newer, better, and hopefully more ethical future in medicine, moving beyond the limiting ideologies strangling healthcare around the world. Stepping back to place the management of critical healthcare decisions in the hands of those on the front line, in clinical practice, not in governments, courtrooms, or academic studies. Above all, clarifying what is often seen to be opaque, impractical, and, at worst, a barrier to adequate healthcare.

When considering "Medical Ethics" and the overlapping field of "Bioethics", one is led to imagine that it is a question of applying some moral category to science and clinical practice. In reality, the word 'bioethics' was coined by a biologist, Van Rensselaer Potter, in 1970, originating from the foresight that it was necessary, in the face of the constant and rapid evolution of Science, to rethink the philosophical and ethical categories which traditionally reined in this progress to prevent gross abuse. Many years later, we can appreciate how correct that intuition was. In point of fact, we have long been dragged toward the future by a Scientific Method that seems unstoppable. The first in-vitro fertilisation procedure seems like yesterday to the oldest generations of medical practitioners, and yet today, we already face the reality of human cloning and germline editing. In the 1960s, the first transplants were developed, and today we attempt to reproduce diseased organs using reverse-engineered stem cells. Fifty years ago, minimally functional prostheses were fabricated to support persons that had lost a limb. Yet, today we study (and sometimes experience) the intertwining interfaces between robots and human beings and a cybernetic future. In some respects, these prostheses may even be superior to native limbs.

A point of clarity at this juncture, the terms "Medical Ethics" and "Bioethics" are not interchangeable. "Medical Ethics", occasionally called 'Clinical Ethics', is self-limited in scope to the very particular societal roles of healthcare. What is permissible and even necessary for medical personnel to do to another human being for the sake of their health and wellbeing would be criminal in most other circumstances. We are privileged to know the most intimate secrets of a person's life, examine and touch them at their most vulnerable, and even cut into and remove parts of them if medically indicated. Doctors have the authority to restrain people and deny them liberty if they are deemed a danger to themselves and others. Everything documented by the clinical team is taken to be real and true in any court of law, even to the detriment of the patient. The right to experiment on both healthy and sick people is even our domain. We are entrusted with the discretion to act, and legal powers back our decisions. This is the focus of this work.

"Bioethics" on the other hand, encompasses a wider scope of biological fields, including medical practice to a degree, but also environmental biology, applied sciences and technologies, clinical research, biological warfare, public health, and sanitation, to name a few. The scope of such a field is necessarily broad so as to apply the unique perspectives acquired through education and training to many dilemmas all impacting human health today and in the future. While bioethicists are of unique value in hospitals and academic centres, most do not practice directly with physicians, let alone are practising physicians themselves, and so most are limited in the impact they have in day-to-day practice outside of medical education and policy making.

Today, we know how and what we are made of biologically (genes and molecules), and we try to use this knowledge not only to cure diseases but even to prevent them entirely. And if we are not sick, we try to use these techniques to improve our physical and mental performance. So, this is medical ethics, learning to ask questions about our present and future clinical and related social realities. However, it is also a more complex part of medicine and, in some ways, more linked to our daily experience than the strict provider-patient relationship, essential as that remains.

The value of medical ethics is in the relative objectivity it emphasises for medical practitioners when faced with dilemmas in routine clinical care and beyond. By emphasising the values of medical ethics and using frameworks to approach difficulties in a multilateral manner, the hope is that every practitioner will be capable of not only providing the best care they can beyond the Medical Sciences and clinical guidelines but rekindle the trust and faith in the medical profession that has steadily been eroded over the last years.

Medicine, made up of doctors, nurses, health care assistants (HCA), pharmacists, technicians, and many more, is under ideal circumstances, entirely autonomous from the influence of politics, religion, and market forces. This is, however, not the case in the 21st century and is unlikely to happen anytime soon. Nevertheless, it is in the best interests of our patients and societies as a whole that members of the medical profession adhere to these core values and use ethical reasoning to avoid the egregious harms recorded in medical history from ever repeating themselves. Furthermore, these tools may be essential to approach the evaluation of emerging ethical dilemmas as science and medicine progress ever faster. It is not enough to expect philosophers, theologians, and 'armchair ethicists' to find all the solutions to complex ethical conundrums.

<u>Every member of the clinical team has a voice and should be capable of advocating for patients in a well-informed and ethical manner.</u>

Why this book? There are many other introductory texts to medical ethics, after all. Many are written by prestigious, well-established, even world-famous medical ethicists, philosophers, and clinicians at prestigious medical and research institutions. While the authors don't discourage any reader from exploring other texts, on the contrary, it is encouraged, with the caveat that you should be aware of where and when these texts were written. Most introductory texts are written in the context of the countries and societies they are based in, often concerning laws applicable only in those countries, with possible biases towards the moral norms of those societies and cultures. Most also refer to medical and nursing programs alone.

On the other hand, this book is not written with respect to any one society, culture, or location. It is entirely separate from the context of the place where you will practice. This means that the greatest strength of this book, that it is unflavoured by association with legal considerations and cultural norms, is also its greatest weakness. It is on the individual practitioner to add that context into their practice and their deliberations on the most ethical resolution for the dilemma in front of them within the socio-cultural-religious environment they are practising in. This book also focuses on practical considerations, as medical ethics is fundamentally a discipline based on science, logical reasoning, and clinical utility. However, more philosophical sections are needed to appreciate the 'big picture' of medical ethics.

This book is also not written specifically for medical or nursing students. It is written for all who work within the field of healthcare. It is commonly misunderstood that the ethics for different roles differ as the responsibilities and level of patient-provider interactions differ. Yet, the fundamentals are the same. The aims towards both patients and society at larger are the same. While the doctors may tend to lead the clinical team, nursing colleagues are now strongly encouraged to voice issues and concerns as a parallel team of qualified professionals, increasingly throwing off the historical role of subservient assistants and taking on independent practices and responsibilities in many places. Pharmacists, HCAs, Therapists, and Technicians are increasingly active in hands-on patient care within hospitals and without. All have obligations towards the patient, albeit without the same levels of privilege and responsibility as the doctors and nurses, even today. Nevertheless, with common aims and fundamentals, this book is for all who wish to practice healthcare more ethically and communicate on a similar footing. As such, with few exceptions, the word 'practitioners' applies to all, and 'doctor' or 'nurse' is used only in specific circumstances and examples.

The contents of this book are threefold: An introduction and explanation of the core values underpinning ethical medical practice and some of the scope of medical practice, a description of the principles and duties underlying the frameworks used to approach ethical dilemmas, and finally, an introduction to the many different frameworks that can be used to approach any given ethical context along with examples of methodologies that may be practically useful.

Ultimately, the objective of this text is not to teach you how to be an ethical practitioner per se. There is often no final and undisputable ethical solution to any given dilemma. Often, this is one of the hardest things for students to come to grips with, the relative uncertainty and gradients within ethical deliberations. Unfortunately, this is on par with most of Medicine and arguably much of science and society in this day and age. This very uncertainty may be the very reason for the dangerous shifts evident in the world today, with the ever-increasing polarization of political groups, religious groups, and even activism for important causes. We crave 'certainty' as humans and are attracted to charismatic peoples and ideologies that promise it. These shifts are inevitably affecting the perception of values in medicine, with a disturbing trend in recent years backward towards a more paternalistic, and less patient-centric practice of clinical medicine.

If you, the reader, are expecting a description of common ethical dilemmas such as euthanasia, abortion, genome manipulation in vivo, and matters of informed consent, you will have to wait for future publications or refer to other texts. Limited examples will be given in discussions of the various sections and for illustration at the end of the text. Still, no global summaries of these common and uncommon ethical situations will be found in this text.

This book aims to prepare you to approach ethical dilemmas and to appreciate why the value judgments and Professional reasoning in ethical dilemmas must be divorced from your personal moral frameworks and biases.

In anticipation, it is worth brief consideration of some of the values that are core to medical ethics and by extension, to the practice of medicine in the 21st century. In no particular order:

- Self-determination
- Solidarity
- Respect
- Impartiality
- Vulnerability
- Betterment
- Kindness
- Compassion
- Scepticism
- Trust
- Peace
- Dignity

Most anyone in any society in the world can appreciate these values in the context of medical practice. Practitioners who work to the benefit of all their patients, irrespective of age, gender, or creed, with respect for their wishes, desires, and needs, while caring for their pain and suffering with compassion and kindness. Scientifically minded individuals, taking the best of their fields and critically assessing evidence in all forms to be worthy of the trust fostered between providers and patients, treating disease while promoting good health. People aiming to develop an environment of peace and harmony, which predisposes to the healing of those in need, and trusting that the secrets of their lives and bodies are private, undisclosed to anyone who doesn't need to know. Leaders in society advocating for progress that is equitable, global, and defensible to future generations.

A dream of an extraordinary group of professionals who see their jobs as much more than just the hours they are paid to work.

This dream is shared between the authors and the many individuals who have contributed indirectly to this text through clinical discussions, active debates, and published literature.

The design of this book is to be read in one or two sittings ideally, then referred to for reference or revision later as needed. Short and concise, taking the reader through a very brief history of medical ethics, an overview of the scope of this field, and some modern issues in medical care. This is followed by a consideration of the values embraced by medical personnel and some of the implications. Finally, we will introduce some of the frameworks of modern medical ethics and approaches to put these into practice.

A few cases for group discussion are included in Appendix 1 as well as online resources in Appendix 2 and examples of reputable Master level programs in Medical Ethics and Bioethics in Appendix 3.

# The Scope of Medical Ethics in Modern Medicine

Usually, a section would be included detailing the long and glorious history of medical ethics. Yet there isn't such a section, just this short passage. The record is not so long, and it certainly isn't glorious. In truth, it's a grim series of events, and most of history poorly favours the actions of medical practitioners. From Hippocrates and Plato to the Renaissance via the philosophies of Christianity, Judaism, and Islam, medical ethics was formed from a hodgepodge of cultural traditions and philosophical fields. Most physicians are only aware of the Hippocratic oath, with no thought to the Code of Hammurabi, dating back to 1750 BCE or the Edwin Smith Papryus from circa 1600 BCE. Each of these, along with the Charaka Samhita in India later in the $2^{nd}$ century BCE, form the ancient foundations of what most societies globally perceive as healthcare practitioners.

The foundations of the first "modern" medical ethics of the $19^{th}$ century were codified first by Percival in his *Medical Ethics (1798)* to settle arguments between healthcare workers in England before eventual publication in 1803, then more formally codified by the American Medical Association (AMA) in 1845 in the first AMA Code of Medical Ethics. John Gregory had first proposed his Socratic alternative approach to medical ethics in Edinburgh in 1776 but this was ultimately dismissed in favour of Percival's later model of Paternalism. Fast forward to the controversies of the early $20^{th}$ century and the first mentions of informed consent. Most progress was then rapidly shadowed by two world wars and the atrocities committed by Nazi scientists and doctors in the name of scientific and medical 'progress', and we reach the birth of a new dawn in ethics. A series of codes, declarations, and global organisations were created to prevent those same atrocities again.

Yet, innumerable examples of gross violations of those new norms are well documented, and the same new standards were ignored in the face of scientific progress. Modern ethics, born from theology, philosophy, and eventually clinical need in the 1960s and 70s, was slow to develop and strongly resisted by the majority of the medical profession. More progress in the 90s and early 2000s led to more modern iterations and are well summarised in numerous papers, available as open access along with obligations in law for ethical conduct, government-appointed oversight authorities, and new centres for ethical education globally.

Today, national centres of ethical thought such as the Welcome Trust and the Nuffield Council, as well as reputable academic institutions such as the Oxford Uehiro Centre, lead ethical debates around the world on issues as diverse as genetic editing in In Vitro Fertilisation (IVF), neuro-ethics with evolving technologies, and end-of-life care ethics including euthanasia. Further, these centres frequently advise governments and policymakers nationally and internationally to better craft tomorrow's laws.

However, while such institutions are undoubtedly valuable at a macroscopic level, they are of limited use in a healthcare setting and to the patient in front of you. For this, you, the soon-to-be ethical practitioner-in-training, must act on the precarious balance between provider and patient, using your best judgement. Hopefully, with some of the foundational knowledge from later in this book, ethical dilemmas will become more accessible and less arbitrarily managed. While they provide broad guidance, you must decide what is optimal in the moment for your patient and their unique circumstances.

> *"She should have realized he'd be attracted to [...them...] for their vision of a world that was black and white. Could she have prepared him better? Shown him that the world was not black and white – it wasn't even grey. It was full of colours that sometimes didn't fit into any spectrum of morality."*
>
> *From "Towers of Midnight" by R. Jordan and B. Sanderson*

Over the years, many widely different ethical approaches have been developed in many countries, most of which are included in the so-called 'normative ethics' domain. These lines of action and thought, derived from moral philosophies and/or religious standards, emphasise the values that have been transformed into the deontological norms of medical professions and laws worldwide. Normative ethical approaches are contrasted in this book by Narrative Ethics which places the patient at the centre of the dilemma and seeks to solve dilemmas through a narrative lens, unburdened by philosophical and ideological considerations. These two are further contrasted with other, less orthodox approaches to provide balance and perspective in almost any case.

It is essential to remember that ethics moves far beyond the simple black and white, or even grey, between 'good and evil'. If you must think in monochrome, much of medical ethics and medical practice lies in this grey 'twilight' area, only distinguished from other circumstances by varying, subtle shades. "Good and Bad", "Right and Wrong", and "Heaven and Hell" are polar positions which do not assist us in the understanding of realities and are some of the most challenging concepts for students, or even professionals, to abandon. This is an extension of "boxing" or "categorisation", where all that falls within a given scope is defined as one thing: "disease", for example, and others as "healthy" or "pre-disease". This desire to simplify the world is another human instinct, a way to understand the vast scope of the world. However, reality lies on a spectrum, and categories often fail to be clear-cut or even objective! To give a few easy examples, consider biological sex, human sexuality, and belief in God. Just as there is overwhelming evidence of more than two biological sexes, human sexuality is more than the dichotomy of 'straight' and 'gay' or belief in a God as atheist/agnostic vs 'believer' as evidenced by the many religions and subgroups within those same belief systems.

As such, consider medical ethics to be far more multidimensional than merely right and wrong. More nuanced and more profound than shades of grey. Richer and more vibrant. Each dilemma, circumstance, and group of peoples unique. No two solutions work perfectly in different dilemmas. Experience will prove the truth of this more than this text ever will. There are no simple questions and no simple answers. Only the longest-standing ethical dilemmas have any degree of consensus within the professions, and all debates are long and ongoing still. Where practical, a common consensus is illustrated in the text, but that may not comfort some of you.

## An analogy of ethical complexity with food and cooking

As an alternative to the former simplistic, dichotomous, and frankly juvenile approach to ethical and medical judgements, consider an analogy of sensory experiences. They, after all, are not so mono-dimensional. With only the sense of taste, we have five unique, different sensory dimensions with subtle nuances within them which inform our brains of what we are eating and its relative palatability. Each sense may be a dimension apart, but none stands alone in a given experience. They modulate one another. The same, if not more so, goes for our sense of smell before even considering the relationship between smell and taste!

Like novice 'chefs', you enter the 'kitchen' curious and with only a basic understanding of how 'flavours' and 'textures' can combine to form novel experiences. You know only what you like and don't, perhaps with some preferences towards one combination or another. Through training, critical thinking, imagination, and experience, you can combine many techniques, approaches, and traditions into a unique, wholesome, vibrant, balanced, and nuanced style of your own. Some chefs throw the 'rules' out of the window and create bold new approaches uniquely their own, inspiring others to follow them, for better or worse. Others take those rules and reflect on their meanings and origins to better understand how to build newer expressions of well-trodden paths. Still others, consider the old, established ways to be easiest, simplest and 'tried-and-true', and produce excellent results, nonetheless.

The purpose of this metaphor is to encourage you to choose your path and expression, uninhibited by the self-imposed limitations of upbringing and culture that urge us to simplify that which cannot be simplified. Like the novice chefs in this analogy, there is no one way to approach the resolution of an ethical dilemma, and each dilemma itself is unique. Using techniques or frameworks of medical ethics, either alone or in combination, you can attempt to resolve the issue in your own unique way. With practice, experience, and imagination, you may overcome more and more challenging situations with equanimity and professionalism with an even deeper understanding of the many facets that underpin human existence and society. Each solution may not be perfect or even palatable to others initially. Still, with practice and experience, you will improve beyond the basics to competence, then proficiency and eventually, perhaps to mastery of this discipline.

In turn, you may infer that if every professional is thinking about the problems uniquely, then there will be many conclusions from the same dilemma. This is true, and some conclusions will be more justifiable than others. Where significant discrepancy between professionals occurs, mediation and consensus may be needed to optimise outcomes.

From here, the aim is to highlight the importance of ethical conduct in clinical practice and by the diverse members of the medical professions. However, this goes far beyond the routine interactions you might expect, and the subtle and overt threats to modern standards are underlined. While they may seem inconsequential initially, some, such as the choice of which topics NOT to teach in graduate medical training programs, can have brutally real effects on society in the future.

## From Clinic to Consult

Medical ethics is fundamentally about the choices we as professionals make daily. Those choices made both with our patients and without them affect not only the quality of care from a humanistic perspective but also a social perspective, as well as the perception of us as a collective group of professionals. As such, it is essential that not only is every choice justifiable under the circumstances but is documented as such and made clear to patients and other stakeholders clearly and unambiguously. This means talking to our patients as people who are often scared, in pain and may struggle to understand, which places the onus on us to facilitate their understanding and resolve simple dilemmas.

In those situations where simple resolutions aren't possible or where substantial dilemmas are present which defy the abilities of the individual professional and the rest of the team to find a satisfactory solution, an ethical consult may be requested. Typically, this is not to give an 'answer' or to determine the 'truth' in a King Solomonesque manner but to provide a holistic, structured look at the problem. Usually, this is more objective, as they are external to the clinical team and occasionally can do so with a multifaceted approach. Despite the ubiquitous presence of ethics committees in hospitals across top academic and medical centres worldwide, the 'ethical consult' is a tiny minority of consultations made yearly. Further, the dedicated speciality of 'clinical ethicist' is still relatively rare and niche, usually only at academic medical centres. As such, some of those on the committee may have limited training in medicine, medical ethics or even bioethics. Typical committee members include heads of departments, local religious leaders, theologians, and philosophers.

Occasionally, laypersons are included for a more balanced perspective.

As such, it should be clear that calling for an ethical consult should be a request of last resort instead of the default solution for challenging cases... As such, a well-rounded and robust approach to dilemmas by many different members of the clinical team helps resolve challenges 'in-house'. Such an approach also bolsters an ethics consult by having a richly detailed understanding of the dilemma before calling for assistance and evident clear communication between all parties. Further, as the COVID-19 pandemic has shown, having a well-trained foundation in medical ethics can help prepare professionals in all fields for the rapid shifts needed in adapting to extraordinary demands on healthcare systems and better leadership at local and national levels.

Despite more resources than ever before, and a greater awareness of pressures in the medical field, a few select matters deserve specific attention: Moral Injury, Defensive Medicine, and the Internet. While many other topics are sources of pressure on the ethical decisions made in healthcare, these are particularly relevant today. Little of this will be news to senior staff, but for juniors and student, take care to know what you are going into, and the burdens you are going to bear.

## Moral Injury and Professional Hardship

The abuse of medical practitioners and advocates in society is recurrent, persistent, and often subtle despite, or perhaps even because of, the authority and respect members of these professions are afforded. After all, a tired doctor or nurse has less energy and willpower to resist societal changes, that are contrary to good patient care. This may result from overt sources, such as the infrequent violence against professionals by patients and families, or insidious ones, such as unreasonable training pressures, an imbalanced work-life equilibrium, onerous insurance directives, and unpaid (but obligatory) work demands. Moral injury from impersonal and callous management, legal constraints, mounting lawsuits, and ever-rising costs from insurance companies further beat down those who have dedicated their working lives to the benefit of others. With this multifaceted and systemic pollution of the medical working environment, it can be remarkably easy to succumb to the temptation of a relatively more effortless and unethical practice of least resistance. Of apathy and neglect. To do the minimum required by the job description and nothing more.

This must be resisted at all costs, along with the systemic causes, to promote better working and training conditions, and patient care. Much like the slaves of old, modern healthcare workers can find themselves enslaved by their decency and care, with healthcare systems dependent on their employees on the frontline being willing to sacrifice their health and well-being for the benefit of patients. This is possible through perverse employment structures, management, and training positions, along with the apathy of central and regional governments to the suffering of the workforce. As such, critical care, emergency care and general specialities (family medicine, psychiatry, internal medicine) are understaffed, underfunded, and undervalued, despite being the bedrock of modern healthcare systems. Patients tend to have numerous "specialists" driving care instead of a single generalist advised by specialists, for the former model is easier and more profitable for specialists and hospitals alike. This is compounded by ever more complex medical sciences as well as obfuscations by industry and political ideology pushing staff to super-specialisation, if only for defensive reasons. After all, arguing that an expert in their field is guilty of malpractice is hard when that same person has written many of the papers on that field…

All this, before considering the bureaucratic burdens on staff at all levels, outdated and even redundant technologies still in use, and colossal resistance to substantive change by both senior staff, management, and healthcare authorities. Is it any wonder that staff leave for greener pastures or even leave the profession altogether?

The way out of this modern professional slavery is not apathy, disinterest, or neglect, and certainly not a mass exodus of personnel, but instead a concerted, organised and ethically driven push by many people to implement fundamental improvements at every level of care and governance.

## Politics and law

Over the last century, the medical profession has seen rapid advances in science and technology and the impacts of state actors and legislators in the modern practice of medicine. Historically, the practice of medicine by doctors and nurses was predominantly governed by personal discretion and interdisciplinary measures. Later, with the development of national healthcare systems, such loose rules became more standardised and eventually regulated. Some regulated practices are intended to enhance and reinforce patients' rights and hold medical practitioners accountable when appropriate. However, with more regulation came the opportunity from politicians and healthcare stakeholders to impose ideological restrictions on modern healthcare.

The four main domains affected are abortion access, end-of-life care, reproductive services, and gender-based services. As an introductory text, these topics will not be discussed in detail but highlighted as possible examples among many where non-medical personnel are taking a hand in healthcare decisions outside the formal, complex, and nuanced patient-provider relationship. To illustrate just two: abortion access and end-of-life care.

One of the most polarising issues, the deliberate medically induced abortion of a viable pregnancy, is one of the most hotly debated political topics. While the general consensus of most ethicists, professional societies, and women seems to favour reasonable access to these services strongly, the social debate remains. However, setting aside the contraceptive option of these procedures and medications, the utility of these medications and procedures remains for obstetric complications where the foetus may not be viable, or the mother's health is in jeopardy. Where legislation prohibits providers from giving sufficient care, significant harms are not only possible but well documented. Further, such legislation can influence medical education to the degree that some post-graduate Gynaecology and Obstetrics programs may not even include formal training in these elements of care. Such changes dictate the current standard of care and may impact the lives of generations of providers and patients.

At the end of life, the inevitable decline in bodily functions may result in physical and emotional suffering and a loss of dignity and personal autonomy. It is not uncommon for patients to wish to hasten their demise, either through suicide or simply refusing to continue medical treatments. In cases of particularly severe suffering, some may even request the active assistance of their healthcare teams to end their lives more quickly. Yet, though decreasing curative therapy and providing palliative care is promoted in law, most jurisdictions prohibit the active hastening of death, even in irreversible and unrelieved suffering. The principal objections are religious, with some concerns over the capacity to provide adequate informed consent and the finality of the decision with no reversibility. In those areas where active euthanasia and passive variants are permitted, it is often simply an informal agreement between providers and state prosecutors to allow such practices, despite the illegality, based on medical benefit and clinical discretion. However, this is far from universal. Especially in cases of tortuous suffering in paediatric patients, the ethical obligations to relieve suffering may directly conflict with the ideological positions of legislation, politicians, and prosecutors.

The law exists to safeguard the population from the abuses of those who would exploit them. Politics exists, in theory, to mediate between the many opposing opinions in a population and form legislation on the debated consensus and to achieve the 'best good overall'.

In theory.

That may not be the 'best good' for the patient in front of you. That may not be the best for society in the near future. Arguably, it may not even be in the best interest of society today...

## The Internet Age and Social Media

One of the world's most influential media sources in medicine in 2023 is Medscape, a website dedicated to providing up-to-date information, for free, to healthcare providers and the general public, as well as commentaries on various medical issues and cases around the world. Comments from registered members are allowed on most articles. One might expect considered, precise, ethical debates from a group of highly educated and diverse professionals. The comments sections on sensitive topics leave much to be desired... The conflation of personal morality as an 'ethical doctrine' is common. Political ideologies may be in evidence. There are even instances of personal condemnations and infighting. Not only is this an ugly display but it is within the public domain and sheds light on professions divided. When the professions are uncivil in debate and discussion, will the public not be influenced? When words are knives in the digital age, the wounds may cut much deeper and longer than we may appreciate when typing.

Social media has evolved as a force of immense power and influence on the generations living in the 21st century. The ability to share publicly and privately much of our lives and influence the lives of others was formerly only possible in person or through print, then via radio and television, and finally today via the internet. In the same way, mass literacy and the printing press led to seismic shifts in the makeup of historical societies, and today we are facing colossal changes in leaders and public figures through this new medium. The ethical impact here is the overwhelming influx of conflicting information arriving daily and the deliberate manipulation of that information to cater to the audience and even hold sway over governance and social structures.

For medical professionals, the internet and social media may be of immense utility in data and research access, up-to-date references, and education of both them and the general public. It may be a tool for out-reaching critical issues and highlighting problems. All are beneficial to the profession and ethically sound. However, deeper issues are also present, including patient privacy in the publication of cases on Twitter and other media, public infighting between professionals and a loss of the public's trust, non-critical publication of poorly executed science, the ease of amplification of previously debunked theories and their conflation as legitimate modern debates. The COVID-19 pandemic also starkly exposed the many benefits and limitations of the use of telemedicine services and the ongoing deficiencies of the technologies within the scope of modern healthcare practices. This includes the generational gaps in technological literacy, privacy concerns, the involvement of third-party software as a medium for the clinical encounter, connectivity issues and finally, legal barriers with everything from data handling to prescription writing outside of a formal clinical workplace. And all this before considering the resurgence of anti-vax conspiracies and the misappropriation of these as 'legitimate' public debates in medicine.

Further, medical professionals' global internet use has blurred the line between personal and professional. When we discuss issues online, are we speaking as the morally defined individual or the ethically bound professional? What duty of care do we have to our 'digital population'? As the legal frameworks scramble to address these issues and others, the more philosophical debate of free speech vs censorship for the public good comes again to the fore. As may be evident from this text, there is no black-and-white answer here, not even a grey. These issues are actively being debated and considered by professional societies, local and national governments, and transnational entities to provide some clarity. What is evident, however, is that the relative benefits and harms of this technology and other future technologies far outstrip the abilities of governments to legislate. This includes injury to both mental and physical health and has a disproportionate influence over the health of global populations in evolving ways.

From a simple ethical perspective, our advice would be to have a genuinely separate personal social media identity from your professional identity online if you have strong moral positions and a desire to share them. Further, consider that everything you post online can return as a reflection on you as a professional in the future, just as your decisions in the clinic must always be justifiable. Finally, when using these tools for public outreach as a defined professional, apply ethical principles and frameworks to your actions and think not just once or twice before posting but one more time again to be sure.

It is easily apparent to see that the ethical paradigms developed in the second half of the twentieth century are rapidly becoming pressured by both a medical profession that is slow to adapt and a technologically advancing world that is outstripping our ability to rely on outside assistance to offer timely, measured, and accurate guidance. To begin approaching these issues ourselves and to have a voice for the future as professionals, we must first understand the values that have brought us to twenty-first-century medicine and the ethical consensuses at present.

# The Fundamental Values of Medical Ethics

To begin this section, a case illustrating some of the fundamentals.

*During the 2000s, a young manual labourer
at a construction site in Los Angeles, USA,
slipped and fell three meters during his work.
The fall caused a fracture of his second
lumbar vertebra and his lower left tibia. An
ambulance was called, and he was rushed to
the local hospital. After stabilisation of his
physical health, it was revealed that he did not
have private medical insurance, nor family or
other friends locally who could care for him.
As a manual labourer, he had moved from out
of state to work in California and had few
funds saved, nowhere near enough for his
emergency care bill, let alone a hospital room
to recover in. He was taken outside the
Emergency Department and abandoned on the
side of the road to figure things out for
himself, with a lumbar stabiliser and a cast
on his lower limb. His clothes were badly
damaged, and he had no phone.*

Ask yourself, was this right? Legally, there was nothing to be done at that time and location. However, morally, you may see this very differently depending on where you lived and were raised. This is a real case, and Dr Francis' grandmother, a former midwife in the UK and, at the time, a Hollywood actress, came across this man in the street outside the ER and took him home. She nursed him back to health on her sofa, as he could not walk for nearly three months. She saw his treatment by the healthcare system as fundamentally, morally wrong. Do you think the clinicians and nurses in the ER thought so? The hospital managers? Perhaps they did. Nonetheless, they put him on the street, the legally viable option.

In this case, the value conflicts are varied and divisive. Even among ethicists, the relative importance of these values is debated. At the core of this dilemma is the vulnerability of this patient. He is unable to walk or even move, let alone work his job, and therefore unable to pay rent, buy food, or even maintain his hygiene. That vulnerability is also found in the working conditions that enabled the fall in the first place, the pay a day labourer can expect on a building site, and a Society with few protections in place for those who may be unable to afford private medical insurance. Further, his treatment is undoubtedly undignified, and he is now impotent to change his situation, and those who provided his care have relinquished responsibility for any continuity of care. In a system where dignity is a luxury with a price tag, those without substantial means tend to be left without.

There is no doubt that this patient would have preferred to be cared for professionally within a structured healthcare system, with access to social support and rehabilitative services to get him back to optimal health faster. Perhaps surgery might have been indicated on his lower tibia and vertebra, but without the means to pay for the operation, that choice has been denied to him by default. Our duty to 'do no harm' is questionable here, as inaction and abandonment are also harmful in the short-midterm to this person, but he is not dying. Still, there is no legal obligation to provide further care. His clinical team have provided the minimum required to avoid overt harm in the form of a plaster cast on his limb and a lumbar stabiliser ("back brace"), as well as ensuring his life is not in acute peril.

Nevertheless, he will undoubtedly suffer further for the refusal of the hospital and state to ensure continuity of care, both from pain and possibly disability, if not peril to his life in the absence of charity. Yet his team did not fight for him or call anyone to assist him. Within that society, the value of a person is arguably in their financial value, either as an investment, a customer, or a resource. As such, there is no ethical call for solidarity with this individual and a collective responsibility to ensure his recovery for the benefit of all.

It is unreasonable to expect healthcare workers to take all who are so vulnerable into their homes or to rely on the charity of those passing by. As a society and as a group of professionals, it falls to all of us to determine which values drive our profession, and as an extension what we project to our societies, as we go forwards and how we may do better than we have in the past.

In this section of the book, we aim to give insight into the scope of medical practice, some of the pressures, both overt and covert, on clinical decision-making, and the fundamental values that are embraced by medical ethics, as well as those that are not. In doing so, the hope is to foster an understanding of the importance of this type of training in modern healthcare, as well as a consistent, systematic approach to managing ethical dilemmas (as opposed to blanket statements and guidance).

# Why you might be a good person (in your mind) but not a good healthcare practitioner, and visa-versa

*"We all live in suspense, from day to day, from hour to hour; in other words, we are the hero of our own story."*

Mary McCarthy

The quote above has been paraphrased considerably over the years, but the essential meaning remains that final statement. We may be the hero, anti-hero, or a complex pseudo-hero, but we remain the protagonist of our story, ultimately wanting to do what is 'right' in most cases. The apparent exceptions to this are psychopaths, sociopaths, and those who "…just want to see the world burn…", who are more prevalent in the many fields of medicine than we like to imagine. Nevertheless, discounting this minority of the population, most reading this text will consider themselves decent, moral people. People you can trust to do what's 'right', 'common-sense' and 'appropriate'. However, no matter how 'good' and 'righteous' and 'decent' you consider yourself and others believe you to be, that may not translate into being a 'good' healthcare practitioner.

Take the analogy of food and tastes once again from the previous section. Each and every person has preferences in their diet and choice of foods. Similarly, each person has a complex blend of values and moral imperatives which determine their moral framework. This may, like their palate, be limited to the familiar and reject anything foreign to the traditional. New flavours and approaches to those traditions may be as unwelcome as entirely foreign cuisines. That is not to say that those who like very specific cuisines and do not deviate from those are closed-minded or unable to interface with others. However, it is limiting. In a vastly multicultural and global world, the ability to appreciate the "culinary diversity of the world" and the wide variety of thoughts, values and approaches is foundational to any healthcare team member.

Furthermore, the flavour of healthcare and the relationship of healthcare to other groups, preferences and traditions is unique and profoundly flexible. The personal preferences of each of us have little to no place in the interaction of a professional with a patient. Thus, while within your society, culture, and traditions, you may be perceived as 'good', that may not be the case in your interactions with others as a professional in healthcare. This can be a source of deep personal conflicts for professionals who are duty-bound to provide ethical care to their patients but whose moral framework may oppose specific treatments and actions. This is particularly evoked in 'trigger topics' such as abortion, euthanasia, and patient privacy. The latter may seem surprising to some outside of acute care, but it becomes a major personal conflict when faced with family members demanding detailed updates on their loved ones.

## The professional in and out of the hospital: can you ever take the 'white coat' off?

While the 'white coat' may make most reading this think of doctors, it applies to all working in healthcare. We all wear a uniform. We all take that uniform off to go home after a day's work, regardless of whether we take some work home. As all professionals, healthcare professionals are entitled to and MUST have a work-life balance. To take a break from working for their mental health and personal well-being. And yet, unlike most other professionals, healthcare workers, in particular doctors and nurses, have knowledge and experience that is useful and applicable even outside of their day-to-day jobs.

To illustrate this, consider three typical situations:
- An ill passenger on an airline flight
- A political debate on a healthcare topic
- Public health campaigns

Where lawyers may ignore violations of legal rights for those who aren't their clients, engineers do not spontaneously intervene to repair newly broken projects that aren't theirs, or police officers do not act when not in their jurisdiction, members of the medical professions have no such limits. We have a duty to act whenever we can render substantial aid, codified in law in some jurisdictions for all applicable professionals. This may be first-aid, basic life support (BLS) or even advanced life support (ALS), if so trained. Most healthcare workers are expected to be BLS certified, and most doctors and nurses should aspire to have up-to-date ALS certification. Even while on holiday or at the park with our children, healthcare workers always have the 'white coat' in their pocket and can provide initial assessments and immediate care if nobody more qualified is present and until they are. A unique profession is ours that transcends national borders.

The classic case for many doctors and nurses is the presence of an acutely ill passenger while travelling, especially during flights or on short-haul ferries. While the crew usually includes at least one BLS-certified member, the presence of a nurse or doctor may be of great benefit. Some airlines have dedicated ALS kits for qualified personnel to use in emergencies, from labour to cardiac arrest or tension pneumothorax. Such persons are more capable than the crew to assess the patient and advise the captain, who ultimately chooses to continue the flight or to divert the flight, in consultation with medical experts on the ground. Arguably, every healthcare professional should be ready to step up in an emergency with an ethical obligation to at least make themselves available should nobody more qualified or competent be present, especially doctors and nurses. HCA's, technicians and physiotherapists, to name a few, all have knowledge and training that is greater than the average member of the general public.

What, then, of the changes to society which impact healthcare? What duty do we have to politics and public debate? After all, few workers are privileged enough to be remunerated for their efforts in public discourse. It is a frequently thankless, frustrating task, with opposition to even the most reasonable positions for the most unreasonable reasons. Yet without healthcare workers opposing trends in law, culture and politics founded on values contrary to patient benefit, complex as those may be at times, inevitably, such changes will be imposed on the healthcare system without opposition.

Should such lobbying and public debate be left to professional societies and unions? Of course not, as those same societies are collectives that may have conflicting interests within them and be sluggish in achieving consensus and issuing statements. Individuals can be a potent rallying point for those without a voice and those who feel their voices are unheard, and many voices are heard far louder than a few. Who will if we won't stand for our patients and those values promoting holistic health? How do we restore the public's faith worldwide if we can't show that we stand for them and their benefit every day?

In the same spirit, recent public health campaigns and the COVID-19 pandemic have revealed the shocking divides in society: generational and ideological, inter-professional fractures and trust in medical professionals and medical Science that likely hasn't been so low since before WW2. Medical professionals have not been immune between conspiracy, political ambition, and easy dissemination of misinformation. For example, over 5% of Italian doctors refused to be vaccinated during the COVID-19 pandemic and up to 15% of nurses nationwide, despite the overwhelming public evidence supporting the benefit to providers and patients. Such opposition within the professions bolstered the misinformation campaigns by highlighting those individuals as example justifications for their beliefs. Similar parallels can be drawn to previous opposition to vaccination campaigns, particularly the MMR Hoax of 1998 (ref) and the widespread opposition to the smallpox vaccine in the 19th century.

Public health medicine, as a preventative means to promote health in society, is ethically complex beyond the evident provider-patient interaction. The benefits are more nebulous, less specific to the individual and more to the collective population; as such, arguments that the wishes of individuals to choose for themselves must be weighed against the collective good of the many in society. Adequate sewage and refuse systems, clean water and electricity benefit all residents, but they cost resources which must come from Society in the form of taxed income and utility bills. Some will pay more than others, but this is accepted as part of the privilege of living within a modern society. The same goes for security from crime, foreign invasion, and social justice. Yet in health, because it is so intimately personal, such lofty, distant benefits seem immaterial and even non-existent despite evidence to the contrary. Some examples of this include:

- The 1854 Cholera epidemic in London and subsequent public sanitation interventions
- The eradication of smallpox and the successes of MMRV through vaccination
- The smoking ban in public buildings and transport

Nevertheless, only by rebuilding the trust of the populations in the healthcare professions, as well as between us as professionals, will further gains be possible and the deep rifts within society be healed.

## The Values Central to Medical Ethics

In this section, the aim is to reflect on the core meaning of a series of moral values that underpin much of ethics in medicine and what it means to work in this field. The following section looks at other values not commonly embraced as values in modern medical ethics but may be embraced as personal values to the practitioner for their own benefit, outside the frame of their professional activities. That's to say that values not expressed here may be worthwhile in their own right but are of limited utility in ethical medicinal practice.

Consider the value of self-determination to begin with. As modern societies, we push hard against paternalistic authority and demand individual freedoms — freedom over our bodies, choices, and dreams. To deny self-determination would effectively make all who seek healthcare at the mercy of the whims of the clinical teams even more than they already are! A crucial component of modern medical ethics, this value underlies informed consent, respect for our patients, and open communication with all parties.

Solidarity refers to the shared value of humanity and our collective responsibility as healthcare providers. Solidarity with our patients, however, and between members of the professions. Medicine overall is in service to the public. Our jobs do not exist without the suffering of others, and the relief of that suffering is paramount. By standing with and supporting our patients, we not only act *for* them but also *with* them — a partnership. Further, hierarchy is something of an outdated, antiquated system in medicine. All professionals have roles to play, making decisions at different levels depending on personal competence and training. There is never a justification for the belittlement or victimisation of a colleague, regardless of role. Every effort should be made to assist other team members and help them grow in their respective roles and foster an environment that others should look forwards to working in each day rather than dread approaching.

The value of Respect seems almost tacit in medicine. Respect from provider to patient, and visa versa. Respect for authorities. Respect for the system in which we work. For the society, culture, religions, and traditions that form the environments *we choose to live in*. Yet respect as a value is more than just the passive acknowledgement of the validity of different realities to our own. It is an active process of engagement towards every person and the elements of their reality. Not subservient, but not dominant to them either. Unlike other professional fields, respect in medicine is not earned by others but is freely given as foundational to the profession.

Safety may be considered simultaneously overlooked and overhyped in modern medical practice. As a value, safety is not only the avoidance of harmful events but the active development of an environment where patients and providers may be free from malign influence and errant judgement. A person who doesn't feel safe manifests not only overt and covert psychological manifestations of anxiety and stress but also physiological responses which may hamper the healing process. A lack of perceived safety can erode the delicate communication channels forged with providers and the effects may be seen for years, and even generations, to come through the education of family, friends, and peers of their experiences. Not to mention the wider world via the internet and social media… As such, making people not only feel safe, but BE safe within a healthcare system is foundational.

As professionals in medicine, we must not be personally invested in any of our patients. The value of impartiality is in the objective lens through which we can view each case. As such, we can minimise sources of bias. Personal investment applies not only to personal relations with the patient (intimate, family, friendship etc.) but also to their socio-cultural-religious environment. It is all too easy to feel closer to members of one's environment than those from outside of it. This is human and natural. It is also a critical pitfall to be aware of ethically.

One of the most ethically and philosophically divisive values, Vulnerability, as a natural state of being and as a value in medical ethics, is on this list for a simple reason: Medicine does not exist without the suffering and subsequent vulnerability of people in society. To clarify, vulnerability refers to the reduced ability of an individual to have the capacity and personal autonomy equivalent of an otherwise healthy, educated and well-informed adult. All people have been, and will again someday be, medically vulnerable unless they have a sudden catastrophic injury that is instantly fatal. As such, it is on us to value such a state not as a distasteful deviation from normality but as a natural part of life to be embraced and alleviated as needed. To reject vulnerability as a value is to adopt a transhumanist mindset to seek immortality and to embody otherwise profoundly capitalistic values, where the vulnerability of some is less worthy than that of others. To wit, rejecting vulnerability as a value enables the commercialisation of vulnerability and the subsequent exploitation of many in society for profit. The global consensus is that this is not desirable for medical ethics, though this debate rages on in academic circles.

Betterment refers to both self, profession, and society. As scientists, we aim to gather further knowledge and better understand the world. As medical professionals, the aim is to collect what knowledge is useful and to channel it towards improving the lives of patients and society.

What else but Kindness do patients expect from those in healthcare? Yes: professionalism, expertise, and proactive action, but above all, kindness towards them at their most vulnerable. Kindness is implicit, though not necessarily covert, and should be present in our attitudes, conversations and interactions. One of the most fundamental values of medicine, it is frequently one of the hardest to maintain. It is easy to be cruel or indifferent to others. Yet, simple gestures of kindness can make all the difference to people. This may be as simple as taking the time to talk to and listen to concerns, asking how they are doing outside the strict clinical context, or simply being present in the moment with them. It is in the small details of caring for a person, recognising that this person is not 'other' or 'them' but is a person like 'us'. In doing so, not only will their life be improved in some small, perhaps intangible, way, but also their communication with you and perhaps others too. Be aware that kindness is not a superficial façade or stock phrase, but personal, unique, and situationally appropriate.

Unlike the value of kindness, Compassion is much more specific. It is the active acknowledgement of a person's suffering and desire to relieve it. Unlike kindness, compassion is overt and explicit. It is a foundational component of each clinical interaction. Genuine compassion requires efforts to deepen understanding of the suffering patient in all facets and target those areas to maximise the comfort of the patient, as appropriate.

Through compassion, more ethical avenues of action may be apparent as well as improved communication and connection with patients.

Scepticism may seem somewhat unusual as a value. Yet, every professional needs to be sceptical of their patients and the information they gather, just as they must be somewhat wary of scientific data, publications, and industry interests. This is all to the benefit of our patients. Critical assessment of *all* information. In the infamous words of House: "Everybody lies". Sometimes deliberately or maliciously, other times innocently or through omission. As humans, we often tend to act in our own interests, and as professionals, it is vital to retain such professional scepticism without overcompensating to jaded or cynical attitudes. As such, never assume you have all the information or that it is entirely accurate when assessing ethical dilemmas.

No list of values would be complete without Trust. One of the most fragile and ephemeral components of any professional interaction, trust is earned through honesty and competence. To lose the trust of our patients is to damage the collective trust of people in society in the healthcare profession. Perhaps only a small degree with each hit, but over time the loss of trust becomes a critical erosion in the ability of the professions to do their jobs. This is perhaps why politicians are so often seen as untrustworthy: it is hard to be seen as entirely honest and competent in the 'halls of power'. Perception is crucial, and approaching each person as worthy of your time, attention, and professionalism builds trust. Ethical medicine cannot be practised in the absence of trust.

As a value of medical ethics, Peace refers to the absence of, or advocacy against, conflicts. As providers, the aim is to work in harmony with the patient as a unique individual—personalised treatment to an individual who is different to us and others in the world. Peace also embodies *peacefulness*, a lack of conflict within the person in front of us. This may be physical, mental, spiritual, or social unrest, with uncontrolled pain being a typical example of a conflict within a person's body. This imbalance of nociception leads to conscious suffering, regardless of origin or neurological level. On a macroscopic scale, the value of peace is in the advocacy of today's policies that benefit the health of all peoples, regardless of nationality. In an increasingly global world, what suffering is inflicted on one people can rapidly affect many, many others in unpredictable ways. The COVID-19 pandemic and the ongoing 2022-23 conflict in Ukraine proved that definitively.

Last but certainly not least, Dignity as a value. A deeply personal and intimate matter, one's dignity tends to vary throughout life. What determines personal dignity is highly subjective and is not for the individual professional to dictate to the patient but for the patient to communicate to the provider. This may be aided through personal education of cultural norms and gender differences in different societies as well as an understanding of boundaries and personal limits. In all cases, however, it means optimising the autonomy and individuality of the patient, as well as avoiding sources of humiliation and dehumanisation.

Faith and belief as values in society are closely intertwined with what it means to be human. Indeed, no other species is known to have religious or otherwise spiritual expression. By definition, however, faith and belief are ideas in the absence of proof. This may be belief in a person, idea, or higher power, but it ultimately remains a personal choice which cannot be demonstrably proven from a scientific perspective. As a profoundly personal expression, it has little value in medical ethics outside of the limited scope of incorporating patient preferences into the decision-making process and debatably conscientious objections by providers.

The value of "Empathy" for medical practitioners was advocated for decades as the answer to increasingly scientific and impersonal medical services. Many training courses still confuse empathic communication for compassionate communication, further adding to confusion among trainees. Unfortunately, empathy overall implies sharing experiences with the patient or internalising their suffering to deepen understanding. The concept of individual empathy is further broken into different subclasses of empathic understanding:

I.   Cognitive Empathy – "I can imagine, here and now, how you feel"
II.  Affective Empathy – "I feel how you feel, and suffer with you, you aren't alone"
III. Motivational Empathy – "I want to help you feel better because you are suffering"

While in very limited circumstances, affective and cognitive empathy may be useful, on a routine basis, these forms of empathy have been associated with burnout and moral injury. The intangible gap between patient and provider is not only for their benefit but also for you, the provider. To function effectively in the long term, we must maintain some distance from the suffering, even as we treat it. Some would argue that motivational empathy is effectively Compassion, but where the line is drawn is in the sharing of the experience and the shift from a professional drive to relieve suffering to a fundamentally personal one.

Collective forms of empathy, such as social and parochial empathies, may nonetheless be of benefit in combatting cognitive biases and health inequalities when appropriately applied. However, while this is of great benefit to the individual practitioner and patients, it effectively boils down to taking an active interest in the local culture, community, and people we care for, especially the minorities and those with complex healthcare needs, and incorporating that knowledge to improve our interactions with these people and their care. Nevertheless, this is usually a personal development matter, as opposed to a professional obligation, especially early in one's career.

Some within medicine consider Ambition to be of great value in pushing the scope of Medicine further. In and of itself, ambition is not contrary to ethical medical practice. However, ambition is distinctly personal and is only sometimes in the best interests of our patients or society at large. Minor degrees of ambition to achieve proficiencies and knowledge, for example, are usually beneficial. However, excessive ambition can blind even the most ethical practitioners to the harms of their actions...

Vengeance is not the same as revenge but a judgement of persons to redress the balance of justice. As persons with positions of enormous responsibility and privilege, healthcare providers may be presented with opportunities to act against some peoples' interests for the benefit of others. Where the motivation or value of the action is Vengeful, this is never ethical. As medical professionals, we stand on impartiality and with a professional distance from the legal systems locally. Despite our relative power, it is not on us to redress judicial inequalities. Simply put, how can we expect our patients to trust us fully if they fear acts of vengeance while at their most vulnerable… from their clinical team, no less… Yet from time to time, we may be faced with convicted felons, an abusive spouse or parent, or an unconvicted rapist, and have the power over life and death, or just the comfort of that person. Despite their crimes and their victims, our obligations are to our patients, not to redress the scales of justice as we see fit. Perhaps this is obvious to most, but unacknowledged biases are rampant. While HCPs may personally dislike an individual for their social crimes, under no circumstances should that ever be manifest in their professional conduct.

Traditions within cultures and societies can be defined as social norms not encoded in law or religious doctrine. Traditions such as the Hippocratic oath or wearing White Coats abound in medicine. However, while these traditions may be a social or professional glue that helps bring people together, where tradition fails as a valuable part of ethics is the lack of uniformity and agreement between peoples. As such, the justification that something must be done a certain way due to 'tradition' is ethically groundless in many cases. Traditions that add little benefit to modern society and are maintained for the sake of tradition itself can be safely abandoned as needed. In those instances where they are maintained, awareness of cultural sensitivity is necessary, but from a patient-centric perspective as opposed to the ethical value of tradition itself.

Perhaps unusual for some, Gratitude is not valued ethically. As providers, we are not grateful to our patients for being patients and, as such, suffering, nor do we work with the expectation of gratitude from our patients. Personal gratification is profoundly unethical, either through communicated expressions of thanks or otherwise material compensation beyond the reasonable fee for services. The absence of such gratifications may bias against such patients and visa-versa when excessive gratification is given. Further, a patient placing their trust in a provider is not a reason for gratitude but a natural evolution of the provider-patient relationship. That is not to say gratitude provides no benefit socially or to medical professionals, only that gratitude is not of value in ethical discourse or frameworks, let alone treatment decisions... Unlike a waiter or bartender who wasn't tipped at a previous encounter, we cannot justify inferior treatment to those who don't show excess gratitude for routine care. Nor excessive care for excessive gratitude at prior visits...

Of all the values in society, Courage is frequently touted as beneficial. Yet, as professionals, courage has minimal value in the field of medical ethics. The simple reason is that providers are not expected to sacrifice themselves or otherwise put themselves in harm's way to do their job. Outside of the military, fire services, and policing, few professionals are expected to put their lives on the line during their work. Medical professionals may do so voluntarily, particularly in exceptional circumstances such as war or public disaster, but we are not expected or required to do so from an ethical perspective. That is not to say those professionals who show remarkable courage are acting unethically. Just that in going above and beyond through courageous acts, they are going *above and beyond* their professional obligations.

Generosity in a material and spiritual sense also has little value in medical ethics. As professionals, we have a job to do. It does not require our generosity to do so, nor is it ethical to be generous, generally speaking. Generosity implies an unequal use of resources beyond what is reasonable to expect for the clinical need. This may be subtle but tangible. Much like courage, generosity from providers to patients may be justifiable, but it is not required ethically. The absence of generosity in both material and spiritual senses does not imply substandard clinical practice or specific harms. However, where this occurs, one should ask not why providers are not generous, but why they are required to be generous to provide adequate care for some patients. Further, generosity to all patients is no longer generosity but now a standard of care!

Finally, Loyalty as a value is perhaps the most misunderstood value of all. Loyalty implies a duty to a person or group beyond what is reasonable, to personal detriment if needs be. While possibly valuable in personal relationships, it is incompatible with the values of impartiality, scepticism, and self-determination. Embracing the value of loyalty would risk patients feeling they were not free to seek second opinions or to question their providers. It would also tend to promote hierarchical structures in departments, damage legitimate scientific inquiry, and question conventional thoughts. Loyalty to perceived authority figures is part of the persistence of humoral medical doctrine until the 20th century and the modern persistence of homoeopathy and similar practices.

## In Summary of Values

Understanding the values underpinning medical decision-making is essential to then approach ethical frameworks for the evaluation of dilemmas. It would be like attempting to cook a complex meal without a recipe or any understanding of the theory behind the dish. Perhaps something palatable would be produced, but it is unlikely to be ideal. The next step is bringing these values into frameworks that can be applied to real-life situations.

# Principles, Stories, Duties, and other ethical frameworks

At this stage in the text, we begin to consider the more practical facets of this introductory text. Ethical frameworks allow practitioners to approach dilemmas in an organised, coherent, and communicable manner. There is a common vocabulary, along with the application of the values previously highlighted as foundational to the healthcare professions. A sample of useful frameworks, but by no means an exhaustive list, is provided in the next pages. Further, each framework is followed by resources to deepen understanding, if so desired.

The frameworks highlighted are as followed:
- Principlism
- Narrative
- Deontology
- The Nine Duties
- Legal & Jurisprudence
- Religious
- Utilitarianism
- Virtues

Each framework is intended to be used in concert with one or more of the others in this text, as described in the final chapter. This diverges from the original intention of the many authors of these frameworks but nevertheless allows for more depth of understanding from a practical perspective in the busy clinic, at least in our opinion.

# Principlism as a Basis for Medical Ethics

The concept of "Principles" in clinical practice, or to be more specific, Principles of Bioethics, has been around since the late 1970s. For many doctors, the Principals are one of the few concepts they remember from their lectures. Some bioethicists and moral philosophers, so-called "Principalists", rigidly use the four principles to approach every dilemma they encounter. Arguably, there is a simplicity to this approach, but therein lies the risk. The four principles as originally described by Beauchamp & Childress are as follows:

- Respect for Autonomy
- Justice
- Beneficence
- Non-Maleficence

The sections to follow briefly cover each of these principles, detailing some of the immense scopes of each. Within the framework of principlism, any ethical dilemma it's broken down into a series of considerations in the context of each of these principles, where violations of each principle are weighed against respect for the remainder. However, this is easier said than done, given the many facets and depths of each principle.

## Respect for Autonomy

Respect for Autonomy is an apparently simple, yet often grossly oversimplified, concept: the patient's wishes, desires and preferences must be heard, and their informed consent acquired whenever possible. However, beyond simply listening to the patient and accommodating their preferences in treatment plans, there are also elements of dignity and respect implicit within this value, though not explicitly stated. Autonomy highlights our duty to the patient, first and foremost, as a person—a person who has rights AS a person, to self-determination of their values, moral framework and bodily autonomy.

The heart of autonomy lies in promoting freedoms and the ability to enjoy such freedoms independently of others. Whether we as professionals agree with the choices of a patient (in lifestyle, habits, or treatment choice), we have a limited scope to advise about the health of their patients based on expertise garnered from many previous patients and medical sciences. Patients, who know themselves, their experiences, and values better than anyone else can, are better placed to decide for themselves whether to accept that advice or not. The question of who understands a patient's own disease better, physician or patient, is an open question in each instance. Nevertheless, except in cases of demonstrably impaired capacity, patients' choices are always to be respected.

## Beneficence

Beneficence follows autonomy as a relatively simple-to-understand principle at first glance: act in the patient's best interests and to their benefit. Whatever we might be able to do, it's not enough that we can do it, it must tangibly benefit the patient and significantly outweighs any potential harm. For example, a drug or surgery that preserves life for a few months but leaves a patient in utter agony for their remaining life is of little value in most cases. The benefit to the patient, however, must not only be considered only in terms of 'clinical outcomes' or DALYs or other empiric measurements but instead in tandem with the subjective benefit as perceived by the patient. A treatment course that may be in a patient's 'best interest' is not beneficent if the patient perceives no benefit from doing so to their life. In particular, consider the over-medicalisation of old age and the process of dying. If patients were genuinely informed and understood what their course of disease would entail, would they really spend as much time and money in therapy? Perhaps not... after all, life is for living, not existing until your last breath.

Some have historically tried to frame beneficence in objective terms that apply to all patients. Still, even standards such as the so-called 'big three' (Life, Health, and Relief of Suffering) fail to be subjectively good for all patients in all cases. Not everyone wants to keep living (especially when suffering unbearably). Others choose lifestyles and habits that put their health at greater risk for personal pleasure and/or societal benefits. Others still choose to suffer in various ways to achieve personal goals or as a personal 'penance'. Actions by HCPs that override patient choice with a view to promoting these standards, called 'Paternalism', must be overwhelmingly justifiable to be ethically sound.

Non-Maleficence

Non-maleficence, or "Primum Non-Nocere", follows with converse considerations: do no harm where harm can be avoided. While commonly taken to mean minimising risks to life and disability because of medical treatments, it has far more subtle applications. Harms are not merely physical in medicine but also psychological, social, and professional. The consideration placed on transparent, effective, and respectful communication is paramount not only with patients but also with loved ones, peers, and colleagues. When a misplaced word can cause distress, inappropriate body language reduces trust, or a lack of attention implies disinterest, a more insidious form of harm is caused. It may not be as easily quantifiable medically, but the implications may be just as far-reaching, even to broader society and subsequent generations.

## Justice

Justice is the most complicated of the principles and with the most facets. Most medical practitioners consider justice an amalgamation of equality, equity, and law. However, justice is far, far more than merely these three considerations. Justice brings together resource availability and equitable allocation within medical care, local and national legal frameworks, epidemiology, and the highly philosophical concept of 'fairness'. Deeper dives into this principle show national and political biases depending on the authors' philosophical and ideological slants and provide rich ground for debate within the literature. For the novice ethicist, superficially appreciating that Justice is about the 'big picture context' of a case is sufficient to begin with: "How can I best use what time, tools, and medicines I have to treat as many people as possible to the best possible standard? Is this use 'fair' within the socio-cultural context?"

As initially complicated and cumbersome as this approach may seem, when used with regularity, it becomes somewhat intuitive. However, therein lies the trap. Each of these principles is in direct conflict with the others. Furthermore, each relies on value judgments which are subjective to the observer (e.g., 'Fairness' in Justice, Capacity to give consent in Autonomy etc.). In addition, an oversimplification of each of these principles, especially the concepts of justice and autonomy, can lead to a substantial lack of nuance and occasionally rigid thinking. Some have attempted to standardise the application of the four principles in clinical practice using the so-called "Four Box Method", where a series of standardised questions promotes consideration of many facets of patient care and various perspectives. While not solving the underlying issues, such tools do enable a degree of reproducibility in ethical discussions as well as evidence of a clear methodology.

Despite these limitations, principlism is a popular approach to ethical dilemmas, especially in combination with other frameworks. It is sometimes referred to as the American Framework, and arguments have been made that, as a framework, it inadvertently promotes capitalistic values.

Other principles in Principlism

In 1995, these four original principles were challenged by European ethicists, with the formation of the Barcelona Declaration of 1996. The original four were criticised as lacking, at that time, precision and a clear emphasis on other essential principles related to European values:
- Dignity
- Professional Integrity
- Vulnerability

Essentially, providers should make every effort to preserve the dignity of patients and their families, work hard to be fair and unbiased in all cases without exception, and value the human condition of frailty as an integral part of human existence (as opposed to a diseased state to be 'cured'). With due credit to Beauchamp and Childress, subsequent editions of their textbook somewhat address these perceived deficiencies, but considerable divides remain.

With the addition of these principles, considerably more conflict between principles is added to any ethical dilemma. We don't, however, see this as a bad thing: appreciating deeper levels of any issue can only be to its benefit if it is carefully considered. Integration of the seven principles with an overarching mission to ultimately relieve suffering is proposed as a compromise and evolution of these foundational principles.

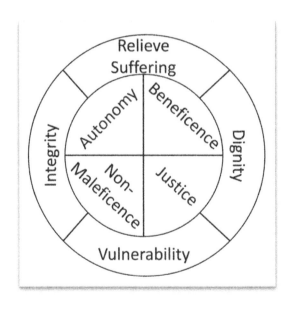

## Narrative Ethics

Often, the regulatory style of medical ethics in normative approaches, such as principlism and virtue ethics, is not enough to help us in our work with patients and families; above all, they teach little about *how* to respect the rights and choices of the most fragile subjects, especially those who are not totally capable or rather are not considered *legally capable*, of making a decision autonomously. These include minors, the very elderly, people with Alzheimer's dementia and other neuro-cognitive degenerative diseases, those with inherited neurological deficiencies and more: people in whom we do not recognise, either by law or by culture, sufficient global capacity to 'understand and decide for themselves'. This is best illustrated with an example:

> "C. is a 15-year-old girl in Italy who has been suffering from cystic fibrosis for some time. She is not a candidate for lung transplantation. She has spent much of her life in and out of hospitals and is getting worse and worse. She knows very well that she does not have much time to live; she has gotten used to the idea of having to die. She is only afraid of having to go through a long and agonising death, as happened to a boy of her age she met during one of her many hospitalisations. Therefore, she told her doctors that she does not want to be intubated and above all, when the time comes, she does not want to be subjected to any excessive levels of medical therapy. Her parents disagree, it is difficult to accept seeing a child die, and they insist with the doctors to "do everything possible, up to the last minute", without considering the wishes of C."

This is a classic and not uncommon moment of difficulty for a doctor and other providers: little remains to be done beyond palliation. The patient has explained what she wants, she is mature enough to understand her situation and to know what she wants, but the local law says that until she is 18 years old, she cannot decide for herself. The law in this case is arbitrary, and similar age determinations can be made in most any country, with a few notable exceptions such as "Gillick Competence" in the United Kingdom (Griffith, 2016).

The narrative approach captures the story of these patients and tries to transform it into a path that the doctor and family can follow. In fact, the best practitioners know how to understand the complexity of life, emotions, and values of their patients. This way, they can make decisions that really correspond to their needs, respect their values and their desires.

Narrative ethics instructs practitioners to approach ethically challenging cases like reading a good book: to learn to interpret complex stories. And like all good readers, a method must be developed and, above all, must be consistently applied. What, then is the character of the patient's story? Who is at the centre of the story? Who should be there? Whose story is it really? What are their roles, motivations, values, and goals in this story? And again, what is the context, that is, what kind of world is being described? What are its characteristics?

The practitioner becomes a reader, but a patient is not a book: they are a person and interact with the reader. How is the doctor/nurse/worker conditioned in their own values, emotions, and perception of themself when they get involved and interact in the story with the patient? And the narrator, the voice, how reliable is it? Whose voice do we listen to? Who do we not listen to, or should we not listen to? Where do the voices conflict?

In the case described above, this is the reality of most paediatric patients; we have at least two different stories, first that of the young patient, with her pain and her choice. Then we also have the story of two parents who love their daughter and would like a different story from the one unfolding before their eyes and within their lives.

The law and most deontological codes encourage us to listen to the young patient but ultimately choose according to her parents' wishes after discussion. Instead, in this case, we can instead apply narrative ethics:

- We can speak directly to the patient in the presence of, but above all in the absence of, the parents. This is because children can feel enormous pressure from their parents and may feel less free to communicate what they really feel and think. This may be from religious pressures, cultural standards, or a sense of emotional obligation to their family members to do as they wish.
- We can honestly share the information we have. Children, much like the elderly, are not stupid. Usually, they need simple, immediate language, but they are perfectly capable of understanding what is happening, and ultimately, they are the ones who are most affected. We must discuss their future, listen to their goals, their desires, and dreams. After all, even with everything we can share, the suffering, joy, and pain belong to them more than to their families or us, the providers.
- We need to explain that we will also be honest in the future, taking what they tell us seriously and in

confidence. We must involve children and the vulnerable elderly in their story, not just their illness. Compiling a medical record, even if very well done, often consists simply of recording the answers to our questions, cutting out what appears 'clinically' useless. Except that a person's life is not a sum of symptoms or laboratory data.

- And we must write down and collect the wishes or even just the conversations we had to follow not only the course of the disease but the understanding of the disease in these patients and to actively remember their wishes when we have to make decisions in their care. Stories evolve with the progress of a person's life, and for this reason, it is necessary to keep the relationship with the patient open and interactive. Indeed, who among us is certain that today's choice will remain the same forever? Illness and disability change our lives, but they also become a part of it, subject, like everything else, to change. More bearable or less bearable over time, and only the person concerned can tell us this.

In short, the provider can aim to ensure that the patient is, as far as possible, the centre of their story and the writer of their story, and to act and advocate for them wherever possible.

# Deontological Codes as a Basis for Ethical Conduct

A superficial, but easy, way to act more ethically is to follow and adhere to the deontological code of the national licensing body you are associated with. While generally dry, dogmatic texts, the core spirit of these documents is ethical practice, though without specific guidance beyond generalised statements. It falls to the individual practitioner to interpret and apply the statements to the case at hand, and as such, it is much like the practice of law. Indeed, statements of deontological codes can often be used as justification for illegal actions in court case, on the basis of professional duty and conduct, codified by the profession itself. However, perhaps fearing similar litigation against the professional body, these codes are often too generalised for specific cases, and may be of only marginal benefit in most cases. Further benefits of deontological codes are their viewpoint on the current ethical priorities of the medical professions, the value of a guiding document to refer to when fighting egregious ethical misconduct, and a reference document to guide clinical practice in the broadest of terms.

Unfortunately, these same advantages also rely on professionals actually reading and learning the codes, some of which are very extensive texts. Further, these texts are not frequently updated and may lack specifics for the field at hand. Finally, deontological codes are generalised statements that require interpretation and are biased towards the culture, society, and ideological context of the writers. It is an assumption that deontological texts are entirely founded in ethical practices, but this may not always be the case. A critical approach to the use of such documents is essential for genuinely ethical practice.

Another approach would be to consider documents by organisations such as the World Health Organisation, United Nations, and World Medical Association. While generally onerous to read, the following documents are foundational to many deontological codes and ethical medical practices around the world:

I.     The World Medical Association: Medical Ethics Manual 3$^{rd}$ ed. (2015)

https://www.wma.net/what-we-do/education/medical-ethics-manual/

A comparatively short and concise document that introduces many themes and situations of ethical consideration and provides decentralised advice for clinicians. Useful reading for general overview and guidance where local deontological codes are lacking.

II.     The United Nations: Declaration of Human Rights (1948)

https://www.un.org/en/about-us/universal-declaration-of-human-rights

30 Declarations of fundamental rights for all humans, signed by most countries of the UN after World War II, with 10 abstaining. This was effectively made law in most countries with the International Covenant on Civil and Political Rights (ICCPR) after 1976, with 176 signatories ratified as of 2022.

Other similar declarations from various intergovernmental bodies have strengthened the foundations of the original document in international forums. These include:

- the European Convention of Human Rights (1953):
  https://www.coe.int/en/web/conventions/full-list?module=treaty-detail&treatynum=005
- the Cairo Declaration of Human Rights in Islam (1990): https://www.oic-oci.org/upload/pages/conventions/en/CDHRI_2021_ENG.pdf

III.    The Nuremburg Code (1947)

In the aftermath of WW2, the Nuremburg trials revealed the scope of medical experimentation on prisoners of the Nazi regime. With the magnitude of these crimes against humanity in the name of "Science" and "Progress", leading thinkers from about the world created a code of conduct that the researchers of the world could follow to avoid similar atrocities in the future. This document clearly laid out the rights of human participants in clinical trials via ten statements.

Crucially, however, it only guided clinical research and not routine practice or non-clinical research, including animal studies.

IV.     The Declaration of Helsinki (1964)

Similar to the Nuremburg code, the Declaration of Helsinki predominantly concerns research practices, but crucially defined the <u>obligations of researchers towards human subjects</u> in clinical trials.

<u>https://www.wma.net/policies-post/wma-declaration-of-helsinki-ethical-principles-for-medical-research-involving-human-subjects/</u>

V.     The United Nations: Convention on the Rights of Persons with Disability (2006)

One of the most recent, but internationally one of the least adopted in full, is the Convention on the rights of Disabled Persons, which demands the equal treatment, medical or otherwise, of all *persons* before the law and public/private services. Discrimination on the basis of disability was to be excluded from society.

The tone and scope of the text has improved with many amendments over the years, but ultimately does not define who/what a person is, nor does it establish the scope of disability before an individual is no longer a person.

<u>https://www.ohchr.org/en/instruments-mechanisms/instruments/convention-rights-persons-disabilities</u>

Crucially, all these documents are not technically binding legal texts, but common agreements that countries that are signatories to the texts agree to implement within their own national legal texts and codes of conduct.

# The Nine Duties of Ethical Medical Conduct

These Nine Duties are derived from the values and principles previously defined and apply equally to all members of the medical professions and should apply between members too. Some are obvious, and others are perhaps less so…

1. **The Duty to Relieve Suffering** – Kindness, Compassion, Vulnerability, Respect, Dignity
2. **The Duty of Respect** – Self-determination, Scepticism, Trust, Dignity, Peace
3. **The Duty of Privacy and Confidence** – Trust, Safety, Solidarity
4. **The Duty of Knowledge** – Betterment, Respect, Impartiality
5. **The Duty of Understanding** – Betterment, Compassion
6. **The Duty to Further Knowledge** – Scepticism, Betterment, Respect
7. **The Duty to Respect the Law and beyond the law** – Solidarity, Scepticism, Peace
8. **The Duty of Teaching & Further Education** – Betterment, Respect, Solidarity
9. **The Duty of Compassion** – Compassion, Vulnerability, Dignity, Kindness

The values foundational in each duty are clearly highlighted above, and though considerable overlap exists, each remains a distinct entity. With a little forethought, each duty is fairly evident, and most are codified in one form or another in law, international treaties, deontological codes of medical societies, and other medical and ethical reference texts.

With this framework, practitioners should consider how each duty applies to their patient's situation and their 'duty' to that care. Where are there deficiencies? What values are being compromised by the current status quo?

I.   The Duty to Relieve Suffering

The first duty of any doctor, today as well as historically, has been to relieve suffering. At every junction, efforts should be made to assist those in pain to find relief and to improve their perceived quality of life. Nobody wishes to live a life of unrelenting pain, and when analgesia is insufficient to manage the physical pain, consideration of end-of-life planning may be appropriate, regardless of age.

Suffering may be misunderstood by some to be limited to physical pain, but the scope of medical practice and human suffering is far broader. Consider the suffering of those with disabilities who cannot function to the same degree without support, both physical and psychological. Even simple issues to correct, such as myopia, may cause suffering due to poorer educational outcomes and increased risks of childhood truancy.

Suffering may be beyond the apparent scope of a doctor's professional obligations at times. Consider the suffering of grief, heartbreak, and hatred. Workplace stress and victimisation as sources of daily suffering and burnout. Moral injury from systematic failures of social systems can induce suffering. Such suffering in daily life can manifest or aggravate conditions such as psychiatric disorders (depression, schizophrenia, substance abuse…) and physical diseases (fibromyalgia, IBS, GORD, idiopathic migraines…).

A frequently misappropriated harm can come from the disclosure of information to an unwilling recipient, leading to emotional distress and suffering. While sometimes this is unavoidable (eg. terminal diagnoses, medical errors, risk analysis), at other times, consideration can be made as to whether or not giving the information to the patient and/or their loved ones will cause more harm than good. In some instances, patients may explicitly say they do not wish to be informed and assign a trusted person as a proxy. This must be clearly documented and made clear to _every_ member of the clinical team. In rare cases, absolutely no discernible benefit comes from the disclosure, or absence thereof, of medical information other than the perception of discharging a legal obligation by the provider. Examples of this include: incidental diagnoses in patients with terminal diseases, repeated disclosure of bad news to patients with cognitive decline, and disclosures to some patients who are psychiatrically at risk of suicide. Where only harm comes from such actions, an ethical dilemma is clear. The resolution of such situations is, as always, unique to the place, time, people, and context. The axiom of 'always tell the truth' is not an absolute, so much as a reliable rule of thumb.

Given these, consideration of the context of each patient in the clinic and their daily life pressures can assist in the management of suffering in a more holistic manner. For many, only with death does their suffering end, and that may be embraced by the patient with open arms.

Finally, a practitioner must not approach Death in healthcare as "The Enemy", but instead as the final step we all take, whether we are personally ready to do so or not. Thanatophobia, the human fear of death, should never be permitted to influence clinical judgement and reasoning, let alone ethical decision-making. Death is a most natural part of human existence, alongside every other variable that defines us living in the first place. Without Death, there is no Life and arguably no meaning to living either. That Life in this mortal shell is finite may be a source of anguish for some but also of peace and rest for others.

> *"To one as young as you, I'm sure it seems incredible, but to Nicolas and Perenelle, it really is like going to bed after a very, very long day. After all, to the well-organised mind, death is but the next great adventure."*

J.K Rowling (Rowling, 1997)

## II.    The Duties of Respect, Privacy and Confidence

Respect is often misunderstood, or variably understood, as a personal quality or choice as opposed to a professional duty. While it entails listening and actively engaging with patients in an open, clear, and level manner, it also requires an understanding of the fragile balance that must be maintained between doctor and patient and the myriad variables that influence each clinical encounter. However, 'Respect' does not mean an absence of wariness or caution when interacting, no more than it does obedience to the patient's demands and wishes. Respect knows no boundaries of gender, sexual orientation, religion, culture, or class but is coloured by each and every one of them in our interactions. A willingness to extend every courtesy and care for others is paramount, as well as flexibility in individual clinical practice and professional conduct while maintaining a professional distance and level judgement.

The doctor-patient relationship is obviously at the core of the duty of Respect, whereby trust, honesty, and clarity can be nurtured from the initial interactions. Not only listening to what a person says, no matter how inane or tedious this may be at times but also **hearing** what they are saying. This is another thing entirely. While much of what is said may be the small talk of daily lives, within this communication comes the tone, rhythm, and nuance of this person's life as well as their interactions with those around them.

Honesty is fundamental in respect. It means not only 'tell the truth' and 'don't lie' to patients, but the active dissemination of relevant information. Medical students should introduce themselves as such, as should the juniors in a medical team. A trainee surgeon should ensure the patient knows they will be the one operating under the supervision of a senior, not the senior themselves. As such, not only can the patient trust you when you say you have said everything, but they can be reassured when you say you are doing everything you can for them. The fear of rejection is never a justification for dishonesty.

Respect for our patients extends to respect for their life as a whole, even beyond their immediate clinical needs, not only in a preventative capacity but in order to gauge the context that makes up the day-to-day reality of this person. To not respect that is to expect the patient to conform to and adapt to the demands of the practitioner, instead of tailoring their healthcare to their life.

Within respect is also the fundamental recognition of the patient's right to medical confidentiality from all others not directly involved in their care. No information about a patient's medical visit, information *confided* in the team, should be divulged to anyone outside of the immediate clinical team. Some hold that this duty is absolute, and any duty to another than the patient is a duty breached. However, some key exceptions are generally agreed upon where the <u>duty to the public and/or patient</u> outweighs our duty to privacy: to preserve the life of the patient or another person in *immediate mortal peril*; to advise the public health authority of a case of a *lethal* infectious disease; on formal requests by the local judiciary and detailed in law; at the explicit request of the patient; in cases of insufficient capacity to provide informed consent when another person is empowered to make a decision on the patient's behalf. This is further expanded in the chapter on the ethics of privacy in medicine.

Respect, however, extends beyond this interaction to interactions with peers, superiors, and the wider community. At no point should a patient ever be mocked or otherwise disparaged. While obvious, it is an often-forgotten detail and the old saying that "...the walls have ears" not only applies to those who are affected but those around them and the patients themselves. Consider the corrosive harms caused by communities aware that their doctors may be mocking them behind their backs. Why should trust be given then? With the duty to silence, discretion, confidentiality and precious trust, lapses in respect for patients and relatives of patients are disturbingly common.

This also applies to colleagues and peers, both doctors and nurses alike. Today, the medical and nursing branches do not operate as a pyramidal hierarchy but as twin towers of patient care with distinctly different, though overlapping, responsibilities. Specialist nursing staff are a font of expert insight and experience and should never be disregarded for their title and role. Cultures of sexism, racism, victimisation, and humiliation similarly have no place in the duty of respect owed between professionals.

III.    The Duty of Knowledge

It is apparent that science and learning are continual processes that are never-ending. Long gone are the days when a medical education could encompass much, if not all, of the knowledge accumulated at the time with a few years of study. With the advent of the internet and widespread literacy in English, the acquisition of knowledge has never been easier. Arguably, any layperson can obtain the equivalent scientific fluency in a medical field as a medical professional with just the resources readily available online for free or for purchase in medical bookstores. John Gregory's Socratic vision of a medical field that is continuously justifiable to an educated public is within reach, in contrast to the ever-declining Percivalian vision of the Doctor possessing the authority and hidden knowledge of his craft.

The medical practitioner must strive not only for excellence within their field of practice but to be updated and educated continuously. Learning not only from other medical professionals but patients and providers on how to better serve the populations we dedicate our lives to. Not only people in medicine have access to Science after all. This does not detract from the in-person training and experience gained from years of practice, but on the contrary, reinforces its importance. The only thing truly separating the general public from medical professionals is this and the duties taken upon ourselves, not the knowledge itself.

Beyond the obligations to Science, a practitioner does not work within a bubble of scientific prowess but the complicated real world. Human beings are each unique, and no amount of scientific study can take away from the scope of human culture and history. The duty of knowledge extends to learning more about everything that affects the interaction with patients and the ability to care for a given patient, including a working understanding of the religions, cultures, and traditions of the populations the physician is treating, as appropriate.

IV.    The Duty of Understanding

Knowledge is a valuable thing but is useless without understanding. A computer can store far more knowledge, word for word, number for number, than the vast majority of human beings. So can a library of books or scrolls. However, without an understanding of the *meaning* of the knowledge in context, it may as well stay in that repository for all the good it can do.

This applies not only to Science but also to the doctor-patient interaction. "Listening" is not the same thing as "Hearing". The former is merely the acquisition of information, whereas the latter implies an appreciation of the nuances in tone, body language, word choice, articulation and context. Understanding comes from the acquisition of information, contextualisation, and rationalisation of meaning from what has been gathered. Only human beings can do this (though other animals evidence this in varying capacities), and ultimately, this is what will limit the utility of artificial intelligence in healthcare and beyond. A machine doesn't "think" but calculates probabilities. A number on its own is meaningless, as is a statistic without context. As such, the responsibility of assigning meaning to a given variable or other output is ultimately that of a human being. Even the most powerful AI systems rely on human programmers and/or historical human data to determine decision thresholds. In this case, the healthcare provider is obligated to take responsibility to Understand the information in front of them and putting it in the clinical context. This includes a critical and sceptical approach to scientific study and research publications.

The basis of the appeal of a real, human physician, as opposed to a computer algorithm that may be more accurate at predicting a given pathology with the same data, is the compassion and essential connection that can be made between provider and patient. An understanding beyond the words uttered and written, and as intangible as the air around us, but just as present and forceful at times.

V.    The Duty to Further Knowledge

As a duty, the continual learning and adaption of clinical practice to evolving understanding is a tacit part of medicine, but a doctor's duty goes beyond the scope of current scientific knowledge and an obligation to consider more than just the next set of clinical guidelines, but to actively research, analyse, critique, and engage in the debates over the progression of medicine. All doctors have a duty to lend their experience and knowledge to the advancement of global practice, even those who work in general practice. Consider that it was a general practitioner, not a fertility expert, who first successfully achieved in vitro fertilisation in 1987!

This is also not limited to the progression of science and healthcare but to the wider healthcare systems and society at large. Doctors have a duty to engage and lobby on behalf of their patients to ever increase the standards of care and quality of life. This may be taken further as a duty to engage in journalism, public health fields, and politics.

VI.    The Duty to Respect the Law and to see Beyond the Limits of the Law

Laws, as social contracts and agreements codified by societies throughout human history, have been a fulcrum of change and progress for humanity. With ever-evolving societies and the expansion of human populations, rules to prevent overt harm from one individual against another have been developed. Arguably, it is the laws of Men that have led to vastly reduced homicide rates compared to other animal species, even when accounting for global warfare! Nevertheless, it is apparent to all that the Law is not perfect as no language or peoples can fully express the scope of human interaction nor the exceptions that occasionally defy the words of the law.

Laws are ideally in place to protect citizens and residents and to enable economic prosperity and development for all. While this is evidently not the case in all countries and communities, open defiance and anarchy is certainly not an advisable course of action for medical personnel. Respecting the Law of the land one lives in and the limitations defined is part of being a member of a community and a good citizen. Within a global world, arguably, if a person opposes the laws of their country of residence strongly enough, creative means to leave and find work elsewhere are usually possible.

However, while the law is different in each country, Medicine remains the same. Bound by ethics and deontology, and informed by science, logic and reason, the obligations of the practitioner to their patient may, at times, directly contradict the edicts of the law where you practices. Consider that the legal definitions of "Time of Death" in different countries are not uniform. Whether a person is legally alive or dead may be a geographical distinction, not a medical one! Similarly, while homicide laws explicitly forbid the intentioned termination of a person's life in palliative care and intensive care, this may be the most humane course of action for those in unbearable suffering. Additionally, while a person has a legal <u>right to live</u>, no jurisdictions at publication have more than a case law basis for a **right to die**. In most places, the act of suicide is 'self-murder' and is illegal but simply not prosecuted. Instead, where the attempt is survived, it is deferred to medical personnel as evidence of mental instability and with a legal obligation to 'protect the person from themselves'.

Such fallacies and limitations expose the limits of the law when applied to healthcare. The law is ever a blunt instrument that ideally aims to produce gross benefits with limited harms. In managing the health of individuals, those caught in the harms induced by the law may require creative interventions to limit or oppose this.

Furthermore, as the pace of Science rapidly outstrips the placid pace of ethical consideration, debate, and discussion, so too does Science far outstrip the political arenas of democracies, which are often advised by the preceding ethical debates. Consequently, for many evolving facets of medicine, the absence of laws, as well as ambiguities within existing laws, make for a great degree of uncertainty. Just because something is not explicitly illegal doesn't necessarily justify the act being done, even with the informed consent of the patient.

## VII.    The Duty of Teaching & Furthering Education

As bastions of knowledge and understanding, healthcare professionals have a duty to teach one another and their patients. Within teaching institutions and beyond, the uniformity of knowledge and understanding is humanly patchy and variable. Continuous education of ourselves and each other, regardless of title and perceived prestige, is essential for ongoing development.

Education is ever the most valuable tool in preventative medicine at all levels. In educating our patients and communicating the realities of their care, practitioners can aim to improve not only the health of their patients but also their life and community.

Perhaps of equal importance is the need to educate peers and be educated by those same peers. We will never be experts on all topics, and gaps will always exist. However, if you can accurately understand the results of an exam before calling for a consult, you can more readily advocate for your patient and ensure best practices and optimal outcomes. Furthermore, this duty extends to other members of the healthcare team. All who care for patients should be offered whatever information and knowledge is available to enable them to provide better care. While the job descriptions vary, the allied healthcare members all have the same goals.

## VIII.    The Duty of Compassion

While empathy in medicine is widely recognised as a major cause of burnout among young doctors, compassion stands apart as a professional value that is not damaging. The difference lies predominantly in the lack of internalisation of the patient's suffering though there is active recognition of that suffering and explicit intent to alleviate it. Remaining compassionate is ever a challenge in the field exposed to the harshest human realities. Few laypersons ever appreciate clinical realities, though all expect outstanding care of themselves and their loved ones at all times. Continued recognition and caring while maintaining the professional barrier and distance between doctor and patient is the ongoing challenge of many senior staff who may seem to opt for some apparent apathy at times, perhaps to protect their own mental health. Nevertheless, continued compassion and care for the comfort and dignity of all patients is fundamental to effective medical practice.

Finally, compassion also compounds the duty to relieve suffering when disclosing medical information to patients. Tact and discretion, potentially along with communication tools such as SPIKES (Baile WF, 2000) to break bad news appropriately, are strongly encouraged to mitigate the potentially immense harms caused by a lack of care.

## Legal Frameworks in Ethical Practice

When using a legal ethical framework, the practitioner is not considering just the specific wording of the law in the place that they are practising but also the limits of the law and the spirit with which the law was written, and how it has been interpreted in common law cases. These limits are then put into the context of the clinical case at hand, and consideration of the limits or leeway that the practitioner has with respect to the law is evaluated. It is essential to consider, when considering the use of a legal ethical framework, that most jurisdictions, if not all, have ethical exemptions codified. This "allows" medical practitioners to break the law if there is an overwhelmingly justifiable ethical basis to do so. It doesn't protect practitioners from litigation and court proceedings but does provide a legal basis for their actions, where those actions are *irrefutably* in the best interest of the patient or society, to do so. Furthermore, legal frameworks may be confounded by former legal frameworks, transnational frameworks, and international treaties and declarations such as the international declaration of human rights.

The use of legal ethical frameworks in isolation is akin to hiding behind the law. It IS important to remember that the law is written by politicians and public servants as "constitutional law" or equivalent texts, and as such, is biased and flawed from its inception to the interests of the authors and their socio-religious-cultural biases. Those laws are modified by decisions made by judges at different levels of the courts, "common law" or equivalents, which may reflect the personal opinions and philosophies of the judges involved. Finally, some countries have afforded legality to secular and traditional codes of law, with further nuance and potential biases. While legal scholars and lawyers we'll argue that in different jurisdictions, these concepts have different names and different subtleties, it is safe to say that no one person or peoples within most countries define the totality of the legal system. As such, even within the rigid letter of the law, there is some room to manoeuvre and to try and do the best we can for our patients, even when the absolute word of the law may act against the best interests of the patient. This may require creative thinking and judicious consultation of legal experts to achieve the best outcomes.

To be absolutely clear, we are not advocating for medical practitioners to routinely break the law where they practice, but instead to understand the limits of the law and where those laws don't serve the interests of your patients. Use your own judgement in deciding what the best course of action is, as well as, at times, what you can live with doing, as uncomfortable as that may be at times. Nevertheless, we quote the Medical Ethics Manual (2015) from the WMA:

> *"...often ethics prescribes higher standards of behaviour than does the law, and occasionally ethics requires that physicians disobey laws that demand unethical behaviour" (World Medical Association, 2015)*

A 'theoretical' example of this could be the deliberate overdosing of opioids and narcoleptics in patients with a terminal respiratory disease who are on ventilators. With no ability to stop their own suffering and their death assured, some physicians may facilitate the end-of-life process to ease the inevitable passing of patients. Essentially active euthanasia: which is illegal in most countries.

Yet, numerous surveys have indicated that this practice is widespread globally and even desirable by some terminal patients, despite being illegal. Even in Holland, where active euthanasia has been permissible for over a generation, it remains technically illegal. Physicians are protected only by an informal accord between the Ministry of Health and the Ministry of Justice to not pursue criminal convictions in cases with valid informed consent that follow strict protocols...

## Religious Considerations in Medical Ethics

Just as there is a place for religion within society, there is a place for religion within the considerations in some ethical dilemmas. In particular, this applies to patients and local cultures that have very strong religious convictions and practitioners that may have lines they are unwilling to cross in their practices. It is usually a mistake to disregard the religious convictions of a patient and/or the social circumstances surrounding a case. A classic example is the use of blood transfusions with Jehovah's Witnesses. These individuals consider the use of blood transfusions to be fundamentally against their bodily autonomy, and the use of these products in these patients can be considered an ethical violation if given against their will. Another example could be the use of porcine-derived products in strict Muslims and Jews or bovine products for Hindus. Such products include some biological heart valves and medications used in emergencies.

Many religions have codes of conduct that practitioners are expected to follow, and it is prudent for medical practitioners to educate themselves to be able to respect the wishes and beliefs of their patients and accommodate them as much as is practically possible. Most religions, even the strictest, make exceptions for lifesaving treatment. However, the moral injury to the individual patient may be significant if not carefully approached.

In cases and circumstances where religious considerations may produce ethical dilemmas and other conflicts, it is prudent to proactively discuss the topic with local members of the faith, in particular local leaders and stakeholders, to ensure they thoroughly understand the situation and gain their unique perspectives and insights, as well as collaboration in communicating with the patient and family. In doing so, however, be very careful not to breach confidentiality in any way without the explicit consent of the patient and other stakeholders.

Religious frameworks are also useful for medical practitioners with deeply held religious beliefs that put them in conflict with professional requirements. In particular, this applies to medical practitioners asked to perform abortions and forms of euthanasia and who may refuse to do so on the basis of "conscientious objection". Whether conscientious objection is truly ethically justifiable is a hotly debated topic. On a simply practical note, the practitioner very carefully needs to consider what consequences for their patient they are willing to live with to satisfy their moral position, and if they are unwilling to do so, to consider alternative paths in medicine that do not put them in the position to compromise their moral values.

To this point, gynaecologists should, generally, be willing to provide abortion services to their patients, and palliative care specialists and those who treat terminally ill patients should be willing to do whatever it takes to minimise the suffering of their patients, including life-ending interventions, when ethically appropriate. At the very least, practitioners within these services should have plans and alternative options in place for those patients who desire services, treatments, and terminations that they are unwilling to provide, ensuring that their patients do not lack optimal care and dignity. Such planning should evidently be undertaken <u>before</u> dedicating one's professional training towards a specific field, as it is impractical to demand seismic shifts in career activities from professionals late in their careers.

An essential caveat to the use of religious ethical frameworks is that they cannot be relied upon in exclusion for medically ethical conduct. The use of these frameworks is to ensure the moral palatability of a given decision to the patient and those around them to optimise outcomes. Remember that patients do not exist in isolation within clinics and wards but also within the societies they live in, and decisions you make may have ramifications far beyond the initial clinical circumstances.

To highlight one particular case, a young girl was brought to an emergency department after a major accident which killed her father and brother, both Jehovah's Witnesses. The child had lost a great deal of blood and required major surgery to save her life. The hospital did not have alternative blood products suitable for a Jehovah's witness, and the treating surgeons, in consultation with the ethics department, agreed that a massive transfusion of blood was the only way forwards, and the child's life was saved. Upon discharge from the hospital, however, the mother and her child were shunned by their local community causing great hardship for the already grieving family and the loss of many of their friends, as well as their community and support networks. Remember: our patients do not live in the bubble of our clinics and wards. While the team's actions were ethically justifiable, little consideration was paid to the broader consequences of their actions and the repercussions for the child and family.

## Utilitarian Approaches to Medical Ethics

The philosophy of utilitarianism which can, in overly simplified terms, be summarised as the "least harm for the most good", can also be a valuable framework to approach an ethical dilemma. This framework considers a series of paths as potential options to resolve the dilemma at hand. Each option is considered then in terms of cost and resources needed, practicality, risks, and harms, before the most beneficial and least harmful or costly option on the balance of these considerations is chosen.

Some philosophers consider pure utilitarianism to be the most one of the most egalitarian and equitable approaches to dilemmas. However, it's easy to see how very human considerations and social priorities may be overlooked in taking such an approach. For example, one of the fundamental considerations in any medical professional is that one life is not more valuable than any other, but some patients are given far more care than others. A pure utilitarian approach struggles to justify the exorbitant costs associated with next-generation therapies for rare diseases or even common diseases that may be life-threatening. Treatments usually reserved for children or young adults are justified weakly as having the greatest benefit for the overall cost as these individuals have the longest lives ahead of them. However, this still does boil down to a valuation of the benefits of prolonging some lives more than others, which shouldn't be done from a strictly ethical perspective.

Ethics is connected to considerations of cost, resource availability, and time. Most ethical dilemmas benefit from at least considering the problem from a utilitarian perspective, if only from a resource management perspective and accountability.

## Virtue Ethics in clinical practice

A somewhat controversial system, virtue ethics challenges the provider to ask whether their actions are 'virtuous' or not. These virtues are drawn from the cultures and language of the clinical team and patient. Words describing virtues are relatively few in English and those describing vices or harms are plentiful, though other languages may find different balances within them.

Examples of questions asked may be:
- Does this [action] I intend to perform make me just?
- Will prescribing this medication off-label be irresponsible?
- Would someone I greatly respect and admire as a teacher act in this manner?

The first question asks whether the individual is virtuous, as opposed to the focus of the second towards a relatively negative virtue. The third question is a comparison against a perceived moral standard of your experience as a professional or individual. None of these is a perfect approach, though all may help to expand on a given problem at hand for obvious reasons. They rely on self-discipline and introspection to recognise bias, or on the perceived authority of third parties. Further, 'vices' may also be virtues in some circumstances, such as 'mulish' or 'stubborn', 'uncooperative' or 'unmovable', or even 'harsh' or 'abrasive' in some circumstances. Finally, given every culture and language is unique and may not be shared between providers and patients, thus a considerably heated debate about which virtues are 'virtuous' may ensue...

## Approaches to Dilemmas

Until this point, there has been no clear means to resolve dilemmas. After all, if a person wants to refuse medical care which may be life preserving, how do we reconcile that decision with our professional integrity and duty to the patient to do no harm, act in their best interests, as well as maintain the trust of others in society? To shrug and say "Well, it depends…" is not enough. To each dilemma, there must be a clear approach in the practitioner's mind on how to resolve conflicts and no one framework is infallible. In fact, the most popular framework, Principlism, is well-criticised for lacking tools to resolve conflicts between equally weighted value groups. Various approaches have been proposed over the years, and can be trialled freely, but four possible approaches are given here, adapted by the authors for an introductory level.

## The 6 Steps Method

1. <u>Identify the *facts*</u> of the case.
2. <u>Identify the duties, principles, virtues, and voices</u> in conflict.
3. <u>Identify the connections</u> between the facts, duties, principles, persons, social variables, local laws, and other components of the dilemma. What perspectives are in contrast, including yours?
4. <u>Propose multiple solutions</u> to resolve the dilemma.
5. <u>Decide which solution</u> is the most ethically justified on balance, or at least is most palatable to you professionally if no obvious solution stands out.
6. <u>Defend your solution</u> against criticisms.

In the six-step method, which has been adapted from "Clinical Ethics Methods and Readings" by Thomasma & Marshall, a solid foundation is formed to approach the dilemma and explore solutions. Once the solutions are found, the practitioner must make a choice and then explore the faults in the proposed solution to be able to defend it adequately from critical analysis. As an introductory approach, this method has the advantage of a clear methodology and ease of memorisation, as well as encouraging students to carefully consider all aspects of a case before proposing workable solutions. It also encourages careful reflection on the proposed solution at the end. In some respects, the six-step method reflects the scientific method: introduction to the subject, hypothesis generation, hypothesis testing, results, and conclusions.
Such an approach appeals to many scientifically minded individuals. It is also favoured by some university professors for ease of grading papers. It may also be a very useful starting point for an ethics committee or intra-departmental discussion of a particularly complex case.

Nevertheless, this approach has weaknesses within it. Just as with any formal stepwise approach, it doesn't encourage deliberation between steps, and nuances may be missed. Furthermore, when considering the 'facts' of any case, such details may be subject to personal interpretation and bias, or even the imposition of one's moral norms as 'given fact'… Examples of this could be: "the death of another human being by another's hand is murder" or "parents want what's best for their child". Broadly speaking, most would agree with the statements, but they are not facts. Instead, they are widely held opinions so engrained within moral frameworks that they take on similar personal weight, but *not* in ethical debate.

Finally, this approach is cumbersome and takes considerable time, which may not be readily available in clinical practice. Consider a dilemma during a very busy clinic; a clinician doesn't have time to use a stepwise approach to collect all the facts, review everything through numerous ethical lenses, ponder connections and propose multiple solutions to themselves and peers while dozens of patients are waiting to be seen. Time is a valuable resource that must be used as effectively and efficiently as possible, especially in the routine clinic.

When time is less of a luxury, and in relative abundance, however, this principal argument holds far less weight, and serious consideration of this method may be appropriate.

## The Narrative Method

1. <u>Build the backstory</u> for the protagonists.
2. <u>Consider the interactions</u> between characters,
3. What is the <u>best possible ending</u> for the story? What endings would still be <u>acceptable to all involved</u>?
4. <u>How can we act</u> to end up at one of those endings?
5. <u>Reflect on the ethics</u> of those interactions and potential consequences.

This narrative method draws heavily on the narrative framework previously described while "keeping it simple". Only the most essential components are retained for ease of use. This approach is most useful for a slightly more experienced practitioner who may know the people involved in the case fairly well. It has little utility in the approach of theoretical dilemmas and snap judgements of rapidly evolving situations but may benefit general practitioners and hospital ward staff with familiarity in their ongoing cases to make quick decisions in collaboration with all parties involved. Furthermore, using Narrative encourages everyone involved to really talk, which may lead to the spontaneous resolution of many issues. At the very least, it allows for information gathering and a better understanding of the weighted values of all involved.

On the other hand, this method is at great risk for personal bias. One is rarely the villain in their own story, usually the hero. Decisions taken are usually for the best of intentions from one's own perspective and are perceived as justified. Furthermore, it requires excellent communication skills to accurately explore the different sides of a case, which is an acquired skill that is infrequently trained. Finally, while the resolution of a complex dilemma may benefit from Narrative, it may also be hindered in some cases by an overwhelming number of competing interests that confound those trying to resolve it ethically.

The "Duties-Principles" method

1. Identify conflicts with the <u>nine duties.</u>
2. Identify conflicts with the <u>seven principles.</u>
3. <u>Act to resolve</u> as many conflicts as possible.
4. Ensure the <u>patient or caregiver is</u> <u>clearly informed</u>, if possible.
5. Clearly <u>acknowledge ongoing conflicts</u> to the patient and other team members for their input and further discussion when possible.

This method is a final, last-ditch approach of ultimate recourse when time pressures or circumstances do not allow for careful deliberation and decisions need to be made quickly. It is also a minimalistic approach for anyone otherwise uninterested in further deliberations. As the authors, we know not everyone is as invested in training to be as ethical a practitioner as we strive to be, and that's ok. At least with this method, some attempt is made to act in a more ethically justifiable manner as opposed to the alternative, paternalistic, old-school approach still prevalent in some regions and practices.

While this approach doesn't dig into the multifaceted nature of most dilemmas, it is hoped to avoid the most egregious unethical behaviours by considering the most core ethical values while openly and clearly communicating with those involved in the case.

## Holistic Integration

This final approach, so named in a nod to the Eastern philosophies underpinning Buddhism and Taoism, aims to balance modern ethical frameworks with Eastern philosophies that emphasise peace, harmony, 'oneness' and the connection to one another. It has been inspired by a shared love for cooking by both authors.

Approach the principles in the previous chapters as if flavours in a meal: complex, intertwining and layered. Each dilemma is unique, with an imbalance in the principles needing 'adjustment' to make the whole more palatable. Instead of 5 dimensions of tastes, you have seven dimensions of principles to balance, layer and harmonise with an overarching determination to reduce suffering. With the combination of other frameworks, such as virtues and narrative as "complementary senses", equally nuanced and important in the overall experience, one obtains an ever-greater appreciation of the whole. By then matching the solution to seek balance in the situation, a resonant harmony can be sought within the discordant principles. A Harmony that is unique to that time, place, and moment.

Start simple and choose just one framework. Where are the conflicts? How are they interrelated? What dimensions are there each problem, and who is involved? What obvious solutions are there initially? Be sure to write down everything clearly, using a consistent method. Next, bring in another framework and repeat the exercise. Where do the frameworks harmonise? Are other details more evident? Reconsider the previous solutions critically. Are other options available? Fewer? Finally, add another layer of frameworks as needed to output a single best solution, if possible. Has harmony been achieved in your mind? This is hard to say only on a theoretical basis, but put your solution into practice, or discuss the solution with the clinical group. What have you missed? Where is any discord in the group or relationship, and what underpins it? If there is no resolution, begin again with the knowledge that you have gained a deeper appreciation of the values that need balancing in a dilemma. There is no failure here, only a process of trial and error to achieve harmony, which may be as fast or as slow as needed in each situation.

Suffering from the same drawbacks as the Six Step Method, particularly the time required to apply this method, it benefits from a less rigid and academic structure. It emphasises the fundamental humanity underpinning each dilemma. It is proposed as an alternative, balanced method which may highlight facets of cases previously unexposed, particularly in highly challenging and complex cases. Initially, this approach may be overwhelming and impractical to employ. With time and practice, the many nuances will become clearer, and the ability to approach dilemmas shift from a burden or chore to a delightful exercise of imagination and ingenuity.

# A note on the appendices and cases

At this point, the body of text and concepts are done. A series of generalised cases are provided with a little context and orientation to start you off, along with links to further resources and cases to consider. Bear in mind that the cases are exactly as written, though perhaps in groups you may edit them to make them more applicable to your local healthcare system. They are cases with no clear "right" answer, but many possible approaches which, with more information and time to consider, may be more resolvable, but not with the information given. Here, the objective is to spur you to use the knowledge in the text and group discussions to take some steps towards more considered and ethical clinical practice.

# Final Words and Thoughts

In his book, "The Creative Destruction of Medicine", Dr Eric Topol, MD, describes a 'super convergence' of novel ideas and technologies that when combined with the 'old ideas' lead to a 'creative destruction' and the formulation of new ideas and practices. This creative destruction is highlighted as fundamentally disruptive and requiring fundamental shifts in our approaches to medical practice. Indeed, many of the technologies highlighted in his book are in common clinical practice in 2023. However, little is said about the ethical impacts of these technologies, what are called technological imperatives. As a theme in medical literature, this is fairly consistent with much of modern medicine. Slow to change and adapt to the changing times…

With this book, we hope to inspire a similar, but ethically sound, creative destruction of contemporary medical practice with you, the reader, as the start. Whether you are a student, nurse, pharmacist or consultant physician, there is always space to reflect on and, hopefully, improve our practices ethically.

Medical ethics is often the least favourite topic for students and professionals alike. It is complex, convoluted and with few clear-cut answers, even in well-established topics. It forces people to think really hard and question the world around them, which is quite uncomfortable for many. However, sometimes, the grim reality may well be that you are or will be practising unethically, and so are your colleagues and friends. Perhaps even the very standards in the system you practice are profoundly unethical…

So, what are *you* going to do about it?

Dr Matthew Francis, MD, BSc(Hons) and
Professor Maria Giovanna Ruberto, MD, PhD

# Acknowledgements

Medical ethics is an unspoken bond between all healthcare workers. An implicit understanding that we have a job to do in caring for people. A job that is messy, complicated, and fraught with uncertainty. In writing this book, I'm indebted to a number of peers, friends and family who contributed to the revision process with their insights, comments, occasional confusion and queries.

Among the alpha reviewers are my parents, Alexander and Philippa Francis, as well as Victoria and Neil Chiverton, for their thoughts and feedback on early drafts of the text. Then the beta readers which consisted of Professor Dr Mark Laher, Dr Yasemin Ali, Dr Elizabeth Lau, and Ms Jessica Beach.

Last, but far from least, my co-author, mentor and friend, Professor Maria Giovanna Ruberto, MD, PhD, who stuck with this project with me despite personal hardship, COVID and a busier academic life in retirement than she had in full-time employment. I'm forever grateful for your wisdom and guidance for so many years.

Dr Matthew Francis

# Appendix 1: Cases

The first cases in this appendix relate specifically to doctors and nurses in clinical roles. With the additional duties and obligations these roles have, in addition to specialist knowledge and skills, the persons in these roles are held by society to a higher standard of care. As such, it may be harder for non-physicians and non-nurses to grasp the nuance in these cases. Nevertheless, consider how you might approach these issues in different places and times.

. . . . . . . . . . . . . . . . . . . . . . . . . . . . . . . . . . . . . . . . . . . . . . . . . . . . .

You are a member of an overnight ICU team of one ICU doctor and three specialist ICU nurses. You have 12 beds on the ward, and at the beginning of the shift, all patients were stable. Shortly before midnight, one of the monitors indicated Mr Roberts, a 72M post-heart surgery, was developing a sustained VT (a potentially lethal heart condition), requiring most of the team to run an ACLS code as per their training. As the team responds, Mrs Shin, 45F with a severe infection, in the room opposite, seems to have developed severely low blood pressure, and her heart rate is increasing quickly. Your colleague calls that Ms Patel, F18 with cystic fibrosis, down the hall has just stopped breathing while on high flow oxygen therapy. With three patients rapidly deteriorating, how should you best respond ethically? Each patient requires the attention of the doctor and at least two nurses for reasonable care, though the presence of the full team would lead to the best outcomes.

. . . . . . . . . . . . . . . . . . . . . . . . . . . . . . . . . . . . . . . . . . . . . . . . . . . . .

Peter is a 45-year-old consultant physician in the ER of a top university hospital in the UK.

While cycling with his team in the countryside, a car sped around the corner, and he was thrown suddenly from his bike into the rocks by the side of the road. His teammates called an ambulance. In the time it took to arrive, Peter regained consciousness and quickly realised he could feel nothing below his navel. Nor could he feel or move his legs. The ambulance arrived, and he was quickly transferred to a nearby hospital, where a CT scan confirmed crushed vertebrae from T10-L1 with total rupture of the spinal cord.

He was transferred to the same hospital he worked at once stable for spinal surgery, but despite the best efforts of the clinical teams, he lost the use of his legs and was paraplegic. Peter, being a practical person, pushed hard with physical therapy to meet his personal goal to return to the work he loved within a year of his injury despite the literature which suggests 6 -24 months to adapt to the situation fully. Amazingly, after 4 months of physical therapy, he is cleared to work again, and accommodations are made to allow him to return to work as an ER physician. The entire ER staff is retrained to accommodate Peter's unique requirements, and specialist beds are ordered to enable him to perform critical procedures safely, such as intubation.

What ethical facets are there within this success story?

John is 64 and he wants to die. He has a very strong family history of Huntington's Chorea after 60 years and wants to commit suicide on his 65<sup>th</sup> birthday. His wife, June, passed away 4 years ago from complications of chronic kidney disease. He witnessed his older brother, sister, and father die from this disease. He has 3 adult children and 5 grandchildren, and he lives alone. He has come to your clinic as a trusted healthcare provider to him and his family for many years, including during the decline of his wife in her last months. John wants to discuss different pharmacological options to end his life as quickly, painlessly and as quietly as possible.

After initially reassuring you that he is entirely serious, he reviews a number of different options he has considered over the last months, and why he rejected each, citing the harm to his family and other loved ones from the most effective and obvious options:

"I could always blow my brains out with my shotgun, but that's very messy!" he smiles and chuckles "...and I don't want my kids to have to deal with that. Better I die in my sleep or something."

Throughout the entire discussion, he is calm, focused, relaxed and eloquent. There are no signs of psychological distress apart from his suicidal ideation and he has not taken any drugs. A physical exam is unremarkable aside from his well-established and controlled hypertension.

"I know that euthanasia (is that the right term?) is illegal here, but I'm not asking you actually to give me the drugs or be involved directly or anything. Just some advice to make sure my death isn't painful and to ensure my family don't take me to the psych ward or something if it doesn't work. I hate the idea of losing who I am to that terrible disease like all the others, and I know it's coming for me sooner rather than later. I've lived a good life, I'd rather go out with a smile, knowing who I am at the end."

The law demands you report John to the relevant authorities for his safety, to protect him from himself and prevent his suicide. Discuss. What is the dilemma underlying this scenario?

■■■■■■■■■■■■■■■■■■■■■■■■■■■■■■■■■■■■■■■■■■■■■■■■■■■■■

The following cases involve members of the healthcare team that are not strictly doctors or nurses and have more nuanced professional obligations. These include various clinical therapists, radiology technicians, healthcare assistants and others. While the healthcare assistant role is used in the cases, feel free to replace this with other positions. Does that change anything in the case for you? If you put different doctors and nurses in the case, how would that change matter? Remember that the case is as presented and not how you wish it would be local to you. They are based on real patient examples from reported clinical experiences worldwide, and similar situations are found in many, if not all, countries.

Consider the cases through different frameworks and approaches.

"Ms H. is a 68-year-old woman with a documented anxiety disorder, currently treated pharmacologically. She has been admitted for elective laparoscopic cholecystectomy after an episode of biliary colic three months ago. Twenty years ago, she gave birth for the last time via Caesarean Section, which was partially botched by a junior surgeon leaving her with a substantial scar on her abdomen and a lingering distrust of doctors in general. She was due to have the surgery at 11 am, but it is now 5 pm, and due to COVID-19 restrictions, she is alone on the ward.

You are one of the healthcare assistants on the team, and during a break in your duties, Ms H. asks if she can talk to you for a moment. She says nobody is giving her any information, she's terrified of undergoing another surgery and feels utterly ignored by the healthcare team. She says she felt pressured and scared by her surgeon to undergo the planned procedure. She wants to know if she should call off the whole operation.

As a team member, you are aware of similar complaints from other patients and a less than optimal track record for the surgeon. Yesterday, a patient died during a routine procedure. The surgeon is arguing on the phone with his partner in his office and has been for the last hour. The nurses are overwhelmed with clinical duties as the end of their shift is approaching.

How do you think Ms H. should be counselled? Refer to the surgeon or nurses? Not your responsibility? Discourage proceeding with the surgery? Protest that it isn't your place to advise in this matter? Or are there other options?"

∎∎∎∎∎∎∎∎∎∎∎∎∎∎∎∎∎∎∎∎∎∎∎∎∎∎∎∎∎∎∎∎∎∎∎∎∎∎∎∎∎∎∎∎∎∎∎∎

"Mr Z. is an 86-year-old foreign gentleman with only a moderate grasp of your local language. He has long-standing, but moderate, dementia, requiring around-the-clock care in a dedicated facility as he has no living relatives nearby. He had a stroke six years ago and underwent regular physiotherapy. Today, he is undergoing a follow-up evaluation of an abdominal mass via ultrasound scan at a local hospital. It is suspected to be an advanced cancerous mass. He is unaccompanied at the moment, as another facility resident has come to the hospital, and only one carer was with them.

Mr Z. asks you why he is undergoing the scans as he has yet to be informed by his clinical team. In the HER, it is written that by agreement between his remaining relatives have forbidden disclosure to the patient, but no reason is evident in the record. Nobody from his primary care team is in the hospital today. He appears somewhat agitated and is uncooperative.

How should you approach Mr Z.'s concerns?"

"You have recently changed jobs and now work at a large hospital with multiple surgical units. Part of the local population is foreign, with a poor grasp of the local language. During the course of your clinical activities as a healthcare assistant, you notice that some of the nurses are obtaining 'informed consent' by simply asking patients or their relatives to sign the official document without explaining more than that it is a requirement. In some cases, you have even seen episodes of staff signing on behalf of competent patients. When you ask other staff members why they are doing this, they shrug and state that these patients don't understand everything, and it takes far too long to explain. Besides that, the surgeons are too busy operating, and it's usually in patients' best interests to have the surgeries anyway.

There is no ethics committee in the hospital, and as the only hospital in the region, there are no other options for patients to choose from.

How would you approach these systematic deficits in clinical care? Where are the ethical breaches? As an HCA, you have no legal or deontological duty to obtain consent as they do not personally operate on these patients. Still, you remain a member of the healthcare team providing care before and after surgery…."

# Appendix 2: Online Resources

Nuffield Council of Bioethics:
https://www.nuffieldbioethics.org/

An excellent site of free-to-access deliberations on the cutting edge of ethical deliberations. An outstanding resource with clear summaries of the larger topics and up-to-date conclusions. An often-used resource by the UK Government for policy advice on various topics, as well as by the EU at large and the UN.


Bioethics Today: https://bioethicstoday.org/

The blog of the American Journal of Bioethics, it contains many thought-provoking articles as well as links to the formal, though pay-to-view, academic journals. Useful for professional development.


Journal of Medical Ethics: https://jme.bmj.com/

One of the gold-standard academic publication journals available. Many articles are free-to-view, along with links to articles ranging back as far as 1975! Medical ethics has come a long way from the five issues a year it started out with and looking back on the language and perspectives in the earliest articles can give considerable insight into how profoundly medicine has changed in the last generations. Today, it remains one of the most influential journals in the field.

The Embassy of Good Science:
https://embassy.science/wiki/Main_Page

A community project for the development of improved research practices with ethics front and centre. An essential resource for anyone undertaking medical research tasks. Not clinical, but a useful place to go while branching out.


The Blog of the Oxford Uehiro Centre:
http://blog.practicalethics.ox.ac.uk/

Filled with unexpected and occasionally mind-bending articles from various members of the centre, as well as students, on topics as varied as AI-Language models, to organ transplantation, to the Neuroethics of non-consensual neuro-interventions. Many are pre-drafts of published papers or copies of the published paper itself, whereas others are blog-style musings and deliberations lacking the prerequisites of formal publication. Be careful not to get lost down the rabbit hole!

# Appendix 3: Further (formal) Education in English

**Some Masters+ level degrees in the UK:**

https://www.conted.ox.ac.uk/about/mst-in-practical-ethics

https://www.prospects.ac.uk/universities/kings-college-london-3852/department-of-global-health-and-social-medicine-15003/courses/bioethics-and-society-44662

https://www.nottingham.ac.uk/pgstudy/course/research/2022/bioethics-phd


**Some Masters+ level degrees in Europe:**

https://www.rcsi.com/dublin/postgraduate/taught-courses/healthcare-ethics-and-law/course-details

https://med.kuleuven.be/en/study/programmes/bioethics


We are not affiliated with any of these programs, but they are simply a sample of reputable options. Many more exist across the world at various academic levels and yearly costs for formal education. The cheapest found, in English, was the MSc from KU Leuven in Belgium, with programs in the UK and Ireland considerably more, and those in the USA, Canada and Australia vastly more, annually. Most programs also consider legislation relevant to the native country and state as part of the curriculum. Few programs offer pure distance learning opportunities.